THE HEALTHY
BACK BOOK

by Astrid Pujari, M.D., & Nancy Schatz Alton

THE HEALTHY
BACK BOOK

A GUIDE TO WHOLE HEALING FOR OUTDOOR
ENTHUSIASTS AND OTHER ACTIVE PEOPLE

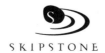

SKIPSTONE

Published by Skipstone, an imprint of The Mountaineers Books
Printed in the United States of America
First printing 2010
13 12 11 10   5 4 3 2 1

Copy Editor: Joan Gregory
Design: Heidi Smets
Illustrations: Kate Quinby
Cover photograph: © Plush Studios/Digital Vision/Getty Images

ISBN (paperback) 978-1-59485-012-7
ISBN (ebook) 978-1-59485-403-3

Library of Congress Cataloging-in-Publication Data
Pujari, Astrid, 1971-
  The healthy back book : a guide to whole healing for outdoor enthusiasts & other active people / by Astrid Pujari, and Nancy Schatz Alton.
      p. cm.
  Includes bibliographical references and index.
  ISBN 978-1-59485-012-7
  1. Backache—Alternative treatment. I. Alton, Nancy Schatz, 1970- II. Title.
  RD771.B217P85 2010
  617.5'64—dc22
                            2009039542

Skipstone books may be purchased for corporate, educational, or other promotional sales. For special discounts and information, contact our Sales Department at 800-553-4453 or mbooks@mountaineersbooks.org.

Skipstone
1001 SW Klickitat Way, Suite 201
Seattle, Washington 98134
206.223.6303
www.skipstonepress.org
www.mountaineersbooks.org

LIVE LIFE. MAKE RIPPLES.

CONTENTS

PREFACE

Not long ago, I was about to give a lecture about integrative medicine to a room full of doctors. Before the talk, a man walked up to me. "What's the point of all that holistic, alternative medicine stuff?" he asked. "Don't you have enough to do with just the conventional medicine? How can you possibly have the time to talk with patients about more?"

It's true that most doctors are swamped for time. When I was working in primary care, I had fifteen minutes allotted for each patient. Half of that time was already accounted for—checking previous medical and lab reports, dictating notes, and so forth. By the time I walked into the examination room, I had at most eight minutes to listen to the patient's story, examine her, and determine a solution. That's not much time for a doctor-patient interaction, as I'm sure you know. Is there really time for discussion that goes beyond conventional medicine?

I believe the answer is Yes, because I strongly believe that no single paradigm has all the answers. Healing belongs in a much bigger universe than just the Western medicine worldview. How can we expect any one truth—

no matter how helpful—to answer all of our questions when it comes to the infinite complexity of human health?

All of this reminds me of the story of the three men trying to describe an elephant. The man at the front said, "An elephant is an animal with a long nose and tusks." The man at the side said, "Elephants are animals with gray skin," while the man at the back said, "The elephant is an animal with wiry hair and a thin tail." Every one of these men was correct—and their perspectives limited all of them. It is only in combining their viewpoints that one begins to see what an elephant really looks like.

The same point applies to human health—which is exactly why it is so important to *integrate* various philosophies of healing and why I now work as an integrative medicine physician. Time and time again, as a primary care doctor, I met people whose problems could not be resolved through conventional Western medicine. It's no wonder that I started looking outside the box. I really wanted to help people, but in order to do that, I had to expand my toolkit.

Which is the point of this book.

Back pain, as you may know, is one of the top reasons people see their primary care physician. Eight out of ten Americans will have back pain at least once in their adult life, and most of the time, the reason is "nonspecific"— meaning your doctor can't quite pin down the reason you are experiencing pain. As a result, we doctors end up giving you pills to take or physical therapy to do—but that doesn't always fix the problem or it may not be enough. Or perhaps you don't want to take prescription medication but you do want to get completely, and permanently, better. So what can you do?

Well, this book seeks to address exactly those questions. In it are some simple, effective techniques to help you expand *your* toolkit in a practical way. We give you a whole host of ideas—from nutrition to acupuncture to yoga to physical therapy to mind–body techniques to stretching exercises—about how to take charge of your back and your health in a way that addresses the whole person, not just part of you. We also tell you when you should talk to your doctor and what to say when you get there. In fact, your new toolkit may even help your doctor to expand his.

This is, of course, one of my hopes. I believe that the best kinds of healing work on our insides and our outsides at the same time—because as human beings, we don't live in an isolated vacuum but in an interconnected web of life. Every time we take a step to integrate different paradigms of healing for our own good, we help everyone around us to do the same. That is how harmony continues to grow itself—and nothing could be more healing for us, or for our world, than that.

Astrid Pujari, M.D., MNIMH
April 2010

ACKNOWLEDGMENTS

In the name of research, I had the good fortune to interview a range of health-care specialists. Our conversations were always chock full of compelling information. Just ask my friends and family: I was always talking about the latest interview. These generous practitioners shared both their knowledge and time. Their years of experience have informed the writing of this book, and I am grateful for their willingness to chat with me.

Two of my sources were an integral part of the research and writing of this book. I lost count of the number of times I interviewed Wolfgang Brolley, RPT, LMP, owner of Stretch Physical Therapy in Seattle. This physical therapist and massage therapist has a gift for explaining how the body works. His willingness to read rough drafts of chapters also made this book a better read. Stanley A. Herring, MD, medical director of spine care at the University of Washington, co-medical director at UW Medicine/Seattle Children's Sport Concussion Program, team physician of Seattle Seahawks, and team physician of Seattle Mariners, took time out of a busy schedule to chat with me several times. An enthusiastic supporter of the idea of this book, he also read several rough drafts of chapters.

Numerous physicians explained the intricacies of the spine, detailing the numerous injuries and conditions that can occur in the low spine. We discussed the complexity of back anatomy; the lumbar spine and the mind–body connection; how they diagnose and treat back pain; and how patients can alleviate their pain. Dr. William Huff wears many hats at Group Health Cooperative in Seattle: he is the medical director for alternative services, a family physician, and runs a sports medicine clinic. Dr. Heather Kroll is the cofounder of the Rehabilitation Institute of Washington, a multidisciplinary rehabilitation program for chronic pain, disability, and a variety of musculo-skeletal problems. Anesthesiologist Mark Matasunaga, MD, runs the Comprehensive Pain Center at Howard General Hospital in Columbia, Maryland. Dr. Joel M. Press is the medical director at the Rehabilitation Institute of Chicago Spine & Sports Rehabilitation Center and the Reva and David Logan Distinguished Chair in Musculoskeletal Rehabilitation. A disk specialist and physiatrist at SOAR: The Physiatry Medical Group in California, Dr. Joel S. Saal, along with his brother Dr. Jeffrey A. Saal, co-developed the IDET technology and procedure for treating painful degenerative discs.

For Chapter 2, "The Mind–Body Connection," I talked with many professionals who work in the pain management field; several of them have worked with patients for more than twenty years. They illuminated how the back and brain work together; how our mind's emotions, thoughts, and feelings affect our physical body; and the role of therapy (and hope) in healing. Again, Dr. Heather Kroll's knowledge informs this chapter. Psychotherapist James Moore, PhD, is cofounder of the Rehabilitation Institute of Washington. Dr. J. David Sinclair is a pain management specialist in Seattle. Dr. Mark G. Strom, an integrative health specialist and medical acupuncturist based in Seattle, is a Tension Myositis Syndrome practitioner. Psychotherapist

Becky Walsh, MSW, PhD, helps people cope with the mental health aspects of chronic pain; she practices in the Washington, DC, area. Dr. Alan Weisser is a pain management psychologist at Seattle-based New Options.

Several movement professionals, from physical therapists to exercise specialists, lent their knowledge to Chapter 4, "Stretch Your Body." Some of them shared exercises, while others talked about how to move your body throughout the day, from setting up a workstation to performing everyday tasks. ACSM-certified personal trainer Sebastian Alery is also a master swim coach and massage therapist. Wolfgang Brolley's knowledge informs this chapter. Barb Mierzwa, OTR/L, is an occupational therapist at Rehabilitation Institute of Washington. Occupational therapist Carolyn Salazar, MS, works at Valley Medical Center Occupational Health Services in Renton, Washington.

I talked with numerous physical therapists, and their expertise informs several chapters, including Chapter 1, "Back Anatomy 101," Chapter 2, "The Mind–Body Connection," Chapter 3, "Common Back Problems," Chapter 4, "Stretch Your Body," Chapter 5, "Finding a Movement Professional," Chapter 7, "Bodyworks," and Chapter 9, "Western Medical Interventions." I need to thank Wolfgang Brolley here as well. Ken Cole, PT, COMT, FAAOMPT, CFI, is the managing partner of Olympic Physical Therapy in Renton, Washington. He has designed a specialized motor control sports medicine program for ground, water, and air athletes for injury prevention and rapid return to activity based on the biomechanical model of the McConnell and North American Institute of Manual Therapy. Annie O'Connor, PT, OCS, Cert. MDT, is the corporate director of Musculoskeletal Practice at the Rehabilitation Institute of Chicago (RIC) and she runs the internal residency-training program for physical therapists at RIC. Mark Looper, PT, MS, COMT, FAAOMPT, is the managing partner of Olympic Physical Therapy of Kirkland, Washington, and principal partner of Seattle-based Olympic Physical Therapy. He has developed a spine stabilization program for both the sporting and nonathletic community. Physical therapist Jane Vess works in the rehabilitation department of St. Agnes Hospital in Baltimore, Maryland.

Researchers Karen Sherman, PhD, and Daniel Cherkin, PhD, conduct their studies at Group Health Research Institute. We talked about their research on yoga, acupuncture, physical therapy, exercise, chiropractic care, and massage therapy, as well as the mind–body connection and the role of belief in healing.

Several movement professionals lent their knowledge to parts of this book, including the "Stretch Your Body," "Finding a Movement Professional," and "Bodyworks" chapters. Stott Pilates instructor trainer Shane Belau is cofounder of Bodycenter Studios, a Pilates studio in Seattle. Valerie Crosby is a certified yoga teacher in Albuquerque, New Mexico. Jennifer Keeler is a certified yoga teacher who runs Yoga Momma at the Phinney Yoga House in Seattle, Washington. Cathy Prescott is a senior teacher and mentor for Integrative Yoga Therapy who lives in Niskayuna, New York. Stott Pilates instructor trainer Kristi Quinn is a cofounder of Bodycenter Studios, a Pilates studio in Seattle. Marjorie Thompson is the lead instructor and program director of Seattle's Pacific Northwest Ballet's Pilates program, PNBConditioning. Seattle-based Laura Yon-Brooks, MA, LMP, RYT, is a sports medicine professional and yoga teacher who has worked with professional athletes.

Although much of the information in "Practices for the Mind" comes from coauthor Astrid Pujari, I also spoke with Dr. Herbert Benson of the Benson-Henry Institute for Mind Body Medicine at Massachusetts General Hospital. Dr. Benson was one of the first doctors that connected meditation and Western medicine in the United States.

The "Bodyworks" chapter includes information from several professionals. Occupational therapist and Bowenworks practitioner Kelly Clancy runs BalanceOT, Inc., and the Seattle Center for Structural Medicine, which are both located in Seattle. Acupuncturist and hypnotist Randy Clere is also a martial arts master, a shiatsu massage therapist, and an NLP practitioner in Seattle. Stephanie Colony, another Seattleite, is a former Hellerworks practitioner. Naturopathic physician and acupuncturist Dr. Kevin Connor works at Seattle Healing Arts. Dr. Lew Estabrook is a Seattle-area chiropractor. Dr. Katie Larkin is a pediatric acupuncturist, an anesthesiologist, and a pain management doctor at Stanford University in California. Feldenkrais practitioner Marsha Novak GCFP, PT, runs Moving Well Physical Therapy & Movement Education in Seattle. Rolfer Michael Reams practices in Seattle.

Along with the doctors and physical therapists I interviewed for the "Western Medical Interventions" chapter, I talked with psychotherapist Peggy Huddleston. Although surgery is a major medical intervention, there is not much information out there for people hoping to mentally prepare for and recover from operations. Her book *Prepare for Surgery, Heal Faster: A Guide of Mind–Body Techniques* fills this role. Dr. M. Pilar Almy, a Seattle-area podiatrist, shared her knowledge of the foot's role in low back problems.

This book wouldn't be in your hands right now without the help of people who haven't studied the glorious human spine, as well. My personal support staff kept me going as I wound my way through the intricacies of both the back and numerous avenues of healing. My husband, Chris, cheered me on, cooked countless meals, and kept the home and family running smoothly. My daughters, Caroline and Elizabeth Annie, made me forget about my computer (sometimes by telling me to "turn that off now"), which was a welcome reprieve. My love of the written word started long ago, thanks to my immediate family; thanks to my entire extended family (Altons & Schatzs) for continuing to foster that addiction and support me in my endeavors. My friends lent their ears and gave me much needed assistance all year long: Mary Fran, Linda, Jen, Beth, Julie, Marie, Kirsten, Dave, my "editor friends," and the entire St. John crew.

Thanks to my editors: Joan Gregory, editor extraordinaire, helped clarify my words and work. Mary Metz saw the book through its final stages. The idea of this holistic health guide series comes from Kate Rogers at The Mountaineers Books and Skipstone. Thank you for giving me this opportunity and walking me through the writing of my first books.

Lastly, thanks to my coauthor Dr. Astrid Pujari. I am grateful for your clear and joyful presence, as well as your impressive knowledge about the human body and holistic health care.

—Nancy Schatz Alton

I also wish to extend my gratitude and thanks to all those who contributed their time, experience, and hard-earned knowledge to making this book a reality. Sincere thanks to Nancy Schatz Alton, who has an amazing gift for distilling complicated information into an easy, fun-to-read presentation. And thanks to you, the reader, for being willing to explore the horizons of this new approach to medicine, which combines the best of every tradition.

—Astrid Pujari, M.D.

INTRODUCTION

MOST OF THE TIME THEY KEEP US UPRIGHT, but sometimes our backs let us down. In fact, eight out of ten Americans will suffer from low-back pain at least once during their lifetimes, and back pain is the number two reason people book a doctor's appointment. (Headaches claim the first slot.)

Whether you believe your backache stems from a rigorous climbing outing, from lifting boxes on moving day, or from bending down to grab the last toy off the living room floor, the root of the hurt may be difficult to pinpoint. The human back is a vast network of bones, tendons, ligaments, nerves, muscles, joints, and connective tissue. Most of the time, we just don't know why our back hurts, and usually there isn't one simple cause.

Almost every time we move our bodies, our back is involved. It allows us to walk upright, to squat low, to run, to jump, and to land after we leap. "The back is structured in a way that allows movement in multiple planes. From the neck all the way down to the lower back, you can bend forward, backward, sideways, and twist, or do these movements in combinations," says Dr. William Huff, a family physician and the medical director for alternative services at Group Health Cooperative in Seattle. A dancer's seemingly effortless series of gravity-defying movements relies on the flexibility, strength, and coordination of her back.

Although you probably aren't performing pirouettes on a daily basis, a healthy back allows you to lead an active life. But when your back aches, you are likely to limit your movements. As a result, your muscles and ligaments quickly become deconditioned. When these elements are weak, you are at risk for further injury.

You know your back hurts—a seemingly innocent movement such as bending over to tie your tennis shoe left you curled up in agony on the linoleum floor. But you can't figure out the cause of the offending pain. Even a visit to your doctor yields no answers. This is not uncommon. Only 5 to 15 percent of back pain problems find a specific diagnosis. Bending over to tie your shoe could merely have been the trigger event in a cascade of signals your body has been sending you. The first injury precursors could have been that annoying ache you experienced sitting at your desk, or the twinge you noticed as you lifted your kayak. Those signals may have been a warning. Pay attention to your low back—even minor twinges or aches could well be a sign that some of its structures are getting weaker.

Although correctly and specifically diagnosing back pain is difficult, easing the pain is sometimes a simpler matter. Luckily, 65 to 85 percent of initial back pain disappears without treatment or is easily relieved. However, although the hurt can dissipate without intervention, it can just as easily reoccur. Keep in mind that these repeat bouts of pain should not cause you anxiety: often these reoccurrences also heal in a timely fashion.

Even if your back trouble magically evaporates, learning how to prevent, manage, and relieve low-back pain is a valuable asset. Americans spend 20 to 50 billion dollars a year attempting to ease their back troubles. Being a thoughtful consumer of remedies is helpful, perhaps even essential, in managing chronic low-back pain.

Although we'll talk about several well-classified back problems, treating low-back pain is not always dependent on a specific diagnosis. The causes of back pain are complicated. Everyone experiences pain differently, depending on anatomy, genetic factors, and psychosocial issues such as life experiences and belief systems. Emotions also play a role. Although your rational mind might tell you that last week's collision on the basketball court is the cause of your pain, your deeper emotional self might tell you that the hurt is punishment for something you did wrong.

Holistic health care looks at all of the factors that affect your experience of pain: the physical symptoms, the psychosocial issues, the rational side of the mind, and the emotions. Although working with a knowledgeable practitioner who discusses every aspect of an injury can be helpful, it's important to realize you are ultimately in charge of your own healing. Whether you experience back pain daily or only a few times a year, living with this hurt is about self-management. You don't need to rely on one system of health care. Medical care today offers a broad range of options: Western medicine, complementary treatments, alternative care, Eastern practices, and more. When you're looking for relief from pain, you can choose from this wide array of healing practices.

Picture the various types of therapies available to you as spokes on a wheel. Imagine yourself standing on the hub of that wheel. You can select any combination of therapies, or spokes, from this big wheel. Massage or chiropractic care might be a complementary addition to physical therapy, or you might use acupuncture for post-operative pain relief.

In this book, we take a holistic approach to healing. First, we'll look closely at the spinal column, learning about each part and how it functions. Next, we'll explore the mind–body connection. After that, we will talk about the back's most common injuries and chronic pain problems. The following chapters will explore various avenues to healing. Instead of looking for one fix, we'll discuss numerous remedies. One or more of these therapies might help you find relief from your low-back pain. We've compiled information from medical specialists, physical therapists, yoga and fitness instructors, bodyworks practitioners, nutritionists, and herbalists. Since our lives move at warp speed these days, *The Healthy Back Book: A Guide to Whole Healing for Outdoor Enthusiasts & Other Active People* offers simple solutions for the time-crunched reader.

The information in this book is based on the research and experience of the authors. It is not intended to be a substitute for consulting with your physician or healthcare provider. Any attempt to diagnose and treat an illness should be done under the direction of a health care professional. The publisher and authors are not responsible for any adverse effects or consequences resulting from the use of any of the suggestions, preparations, or procedures discussed in this book.

1 BACK ANATOMY 101

WE'VE ALL HEARD THAT KNOWLEDGE IS POWER. When it comes to your aching back, this saying takes on a specific meaning. Learning about your back's anatomy can help you navigate your road to healing. Think about your biking trip through rural France. Although it wasn't absolutely necessary to have a working knowledge of French, it sure made the journey easier.

Medical terminology can sound like a foreign language. Still, having a basic understanding of the main parts of the back makes talking with any type of care provider a more comfortable experience. Perusing the miles of online material on back problems becomes a simpler task. If words such as *multifidus* and *nucleus pulposus* roll off your tongue during conversations, people at social gatherings might even mistake you for a doctor.

All kidding aside, learning the backbone's technical jargon will help you create a plan for treating your back ailment.

A MAP OF THE SPINE

Stand sideways in front of a mirror and look at the shape of your back. You'll notice your spine has a gentle S-shaped curve. Now reach behind and run your fingertips up and down your spine. You'll feel a series of bony knobs right underneath your skin. Although you can't feel the front of the spine, it usually sits about two to four inches back from the belly button's center.

The bony knobs you feel with your fingertips are parts of your vertebrae. More than thirty of these bones comprise the spine. Vertebrae are akin to children's building blocks, stacked one atop another with a cushioning disk between almost every bone

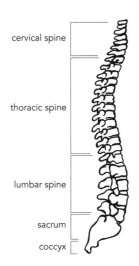

cervical spine

thoracic spine

lumbar spine

sacrum

coccyx

1.1. The Spine

of the top twenty-four vertebrae. This tower of bones divides into sections or regions: the cervical spine, the thoracic spine, the lumbar spine, the sacrum, and the coccyx. The first letter of its respective spinal section, plus a number, identifies each vertebra; for example, C3 is the third vertebra in the cervical spine and L4 is the fourth vertebra in the lumbar section.

The Cervical Region

The head rests atop the cervical spine, which has seven vertebrae labeled C1 through C7, from the top down. Think of the head as an oversized lookout hut atop a fire tower, with the vertebrae making up the ladder rungs beneath it. The bottom "rung," or vertebra, is the largest, with the other vertebrae shrinking in size toward the top of the spinal column. The top two vertebrae in this neck section—called the *atlas* and the *axis*—are unique. First, there is no disk between these vertebrae. Next, the pivot-style joint between the atlas and axis allows for maximum neck rotation. (The joints in our body come in several varieties, including hinge and ball-and-socket joints. The rest of the spine's joints are gliding joints.) You don't really have eyes in the back of your head, but you can turn your head far enough to fool your children into thinking you can see their every move. The rest of the neck's vertebrae, C3 through C7, resemble the vertebrae in the thoracic and lumbar spines, the next two regions of your backbone.

The Thoracic Region

The midsection of the back, the thoracic region, contains twelve vertebrae, T1–T12. This is a relatively rigid area, with the rib cage forming a protective circle for the spine, lungs, heart, and liver. The thoracic region allows for less motion and is not as flexible as the sections above and below. Although back problems can occur here, pain is much more common in the lumbar spine.

The Lumbar Region

Your lower backbone—the lumbar region—forms the bottom of the S-shaped curve of your spinal column. While the cervical spine has a backward curve, and the thoracic section curves gently forward, the lumbar region has a backward, or concave, curve. The lumbar spine section usually has five vertebrae, L1 through L5. Some people have six lumbar vertebrae, borrowing one from the next spinal section, the sacrum.

Likewise, some people have four vertebrae here, with the last vertebra moving into the sacrum. These discrepancies in the number of vertebrae are not a cause for concern. It is normal to have varying numbers of vertebrae and this will not cause pain.

The lumbar region has the largest vertebrae. The weight of the upper body rests on the lumbar spine, the same way a child's building-block fortress rests upon its bottom blocks. This section of vertebrae lets the body flex and extend. A full 50 percent of a body's bending and flexing capabilities arise at the waist. (The hip area accounts for the other 50 percent.) Although all five vertebrae in your low back bend, most of this action happens in the last two vertebrae of the lumbar region, L4 and L5. It's no surprise, then, that these are the two most commonly injured sections of the entire spinal column.

The Sacrum and Coccyx

While your low back is quite flexible, the sacrum contains five fused vertebrae often thought of as a single bone. (Like the lumbar region, your sacrum might also have either four or six fused vertebrae.) The sacrum looks like a gardening spade or a triangle. It connects to the two outer pelvis bones via sacroiliac joints. These two thick joints aren't designed to move much, allowing just a few millimeters of motion. Still, the weight of the body comes down the spine into the sacrum, and then the sacroiliac joint transfers that weight to the hip joint, continuing down into the leg, all the way to the heel. In other words, the sacroiliac joint is an important connection between the spinal column and the lower half of your body.

Just below the sacrum is the final bone of the spine, the coccyx. Also called the tailbone, this bony end consists of three to five fused vertebrae.

VERTEBRAE: THE BUILDING BLOCKS OF THE SPINE

Like children's building blocks, vertebrae are similar in their structure, but can vary in size and in the direction they face. The specific parts of each vertebra face in different directions, depending on the vertebra's locale in the spinal column. Regardless of its position in the spine, each vertebra has a round front part of bone called the *vertebral body*. Between the vertebrae are *disks,* and jutting off the back of each vertebral body are two cylinder-shaped projections of bone called *pedicles*. The pedicles make a bridge to each vertebra's back section and protect the spinal cord and nerves. The *lamina* forms the roof of this back section. Together, the vertebral body, pedicles, and lamina create a protective ring while providing a hole for the spinal canal.

The bony ridge that you feel as you brush your fingers along your spine—the *spinous processes*—rises between the midpoints of the lamina. This is one point of attachment for the backbone, with ligaments connecting each spinous process to the spinous process above and below it. A section of bone called the *transverse process* creates another place of attachment—this time for muscles connecting to the back-bone. Two transverse processes sit at right angles to the lamina and pedicles.

Actual vertebra-to-vertebra connection happens at the *facet joints*. Like the other joints in

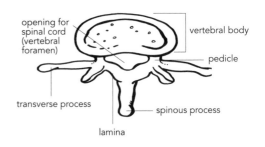

opening for spinal cord (vertebral foramen)

vertebral body

pedicle

transverse process

spinous process

lamina

1.2. Vertebra

PICTURE A BICYCLE CHAIN

The way your backbone moves makes climbing that rock wall a graceful endeavor to watch. Think of the backbone in terms of motion segments. Each vertebra is part of two motion segments. For example, the L4 vertebra is part of the L3/L4 motion segment as well as the L4/L5 motion segment. These segments help your spinal column move in a coordinated fashion.

Wolfgang Brolley, a physical therapist, massage therapist, and founder of Stretch Physical Therapy in Seattle, likens these segments to bicycle chain links. "The vertebra, the disk between, and the subsequent vertebra make up a movement segment. Because the vertebrae move on top of and around the disks, it's very much like two links in a bicycle chain being joined together," says Brolley. "One of the most common reasons for dysfunction in the back is because of mechanical dysfunction. Some links are too stiff and some links have crazy amounts of motion."

your body—knee, ankle, elbow—the facet joints help the backbone move while preventing each vertebra from slipping or moving too far out of place. Think about the hinges on your front door: they connect the door to the frame while allowing the door to open and shut without flying off its frame.

There are four facet joints at the back of each vertebra. They jut out like arms and legs, akin to a roughly drawn, headless, stick-figure person.

Surrounding the entire facet joint is a capsule made of connective tissue. Inside the capsule is a lining, called the *synovial lining,* which secretes fluid to lubricate and feed the joint. This fluid is like the grease you apply to your bicycle chain, which helps the links move easily along the gears and lessens the wear and tear on the chain. The joint capsule creates smooth movement, with the facet joints sliding across each other.

BEYOND THE VERTEBRAE

Obviously, there is more to the back than its ladder rungs of vertebrae. Cushioning disks lie between the vertebrae, making your actions possible and coordinated. Much like undersea fiber-optic cables, the spinal cord's nerves relay messages between your brain and your body parts. Muscles keep you upright and mobile. Tendons and ligaments help you move your body and keep motion in check. All of these parts are interconnected: if a single component suffers trauma, that trauma could affect any of the other components.

Those Shock-Absorbing Disks

The disks between the spinal vertebrae have acquired several monikers, from jelly doughnuts and water balloons to shock absorbers. While these terms can be too simplistic, disks do cushion and support the spinal column. The disks are located in the front part of the spinal column, between the big, block-shaped vertebral body bones. "The job of the disk is to hold the two vertebrae together and accept all of the loads that go through there. This means stopping the vertebra from going too far forward, backward, sideways, or at an angle to each other. The disk doesn't do so by restricting the motion like a solid connection would make. It allows just enough motion, and it damps the motion. So as the motion progressively occurs, it occurs to a slower and slower degree," explains Dr. Joel Saal, a disk specialist and physiatrist at SOAR: The Physiatry Medical Group in California.

Every disk has a hard outer covering of tissue called the *annulus fibrosis*. This tissue actually grows into the vertebrae above and below it. The outer third of the annulus fibrosis contains nerve endings.

Inside the annulus fibrosis is the center of the disk, the *nucleus pulposus.* Often compared to a jelly doughnut's center, this soft interior is the shock-absorbing portion of the disk. This is where the water balloon image is apt. When the spine bears weight, the center of the disk spreads out and the annulus fibrosis bulges, similar to a water balloon after you squeeze it, dispersing the weight coming from the pressures above the disk.

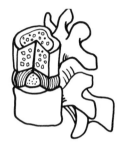

1.3. Disk with Two Vertebrae

The Spinal Cord and Nerves

The spinal cord, a bundle of nerve tissue, starts in the brain and travels downward through the *foramen magnum*—nicknamed "the main brain hole" by anatomy students— at the brain base. Specific parts of each vertebra encircle the spinal cord: the vertebral body, the pedicles that jut off the sides of the vertebral body, and the lamina create a circular channel that protects the spinal cord. (See figure 1.2.) Thirty-one pairs of

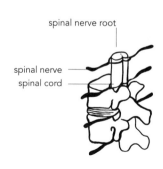

spinal nerve root

spinal nerve

spinal cord

1.4. Spinal Nerves

WHY CHILDREN APPEAR TALLER EACH MORNING

The nucleus pulposus, or disk center, consists mostly of water. During the day, when you are upright, gravity gradually squeezes water out of the disks; at night, when you are lying down, the water is restored. Age also plays a role in the health of our disks. At birth, our disks are 80 percent water, but as we age, the disks lose water content, becoming less flexible and more brittle. Yes, this is one reason people appear shorter as they age. Similarly, young children do appear taller in the morning. Maybe they did grow last night, but they also stand taller every morning thanks to the disks' refreshed water content.

Another unusual aspect of this body part's construction is that injured disks take a long time to heal. Your disks have no direct blood supply. In the rest of your body, blood is an essential healing tool. This lack of blood supply also means the disks age more readily, succumbing to the wear and tear that naturally happens as we grow older.

Moving your body every day helps keep your disks healthy. Disks rely on movement such as walking to receive their nutrition; movement pumps fluid in and out of the disks. Too much inactivity and sitting has a direct negative effect on this remarkable body part.

Here's one last disk factoid to share at your next dinner party: each disk is strong enough to handle loads of up to 1000 pounds in a 150-pound person.

nerves branch off the spinal cord, exiting the spinal canal through holes called *foramen*. These holes are essentially gaps between vertebrae, held open by the disks.

The spinal cord ends before reaching the bottom of your backbone. After traveling through the cervical and thoracic regions, the spinal cord tapers into a bundle of nerve roots called the horse's tail, or *cauda equina*, in the lumbar and sacral sections of the spine.

The spinal cord contains two kinds of nerves: motor and sensory. Motor nerves carry impulses from the brain to the spinal cord and down to the muscles, initiating movement. Sensory nerves transmit messages from joints, muscles, organs, blood vessels, and skin up to the brain. These messages convey information about the outside environment, such as heat and cold, and details about your body's movements.

Muscles

Muscles move your bones, initiating movement and restricting your body from moving too far. Think of your muscles as levers and pulleys, working underneath your skin to make everyday actions possible. Working mostly in pairs, muscles move two ways: lengthening (eccentric motion) and shortening (concentric motion). Consider the biceps muscles of your arm. If you are doing a biceps curl, the biceps muscles are shortening, or contracting, as they work; this is concentric motion. Now you grab a heavy weight and slowly lower that weight. Your biceps muscles are still working, or else you would drop that heavy weight on your foot. Now the muscles are lengthening, or eccentrically contracting.

KEEP YOUR FEET HAPPY

Your foot is the first part of your body to hit the ground, the very beginning of the kinetic chain, translating up the entire leg all the way to your backbone. During *pronation*, your heel touches the pavement, as your foot flexes in and downward to adapt to the floor and absorb shock. Later, during *supination*, your foot rolls outward and stiffens, giving you a rigid, level support to push your foot and body forward.

Pronation and supination are part of your gait, or the way you walk. If you over-pronate, meaning there is too much of an internal or downward movement, this rotates your shinbone inward, which can negatively affect your knees and low back. If you over-supinate, your gait is much more jarring, which can lead to arthritis. Someone with flat feet—meaning there are no upward arches on the bottom of her feet—expends more energy moving because her feet lack that rigid support that naturally pushes her forward.

If you are suffering from a low-back problem, the root of your injury could be your gait. Since any of these foot issues can lead to lumbar spine problems, it makes sense to have a professional look at your gait. Your doctor can watch you walk, but he may send you to a podiatrist for further analysis. Orthotics (inserts for your shoes) are often the solution for gait issues.

Sometimes the orthotics will need to be custom-made. Often,

though, your regular doctor or a podiatrist will suggest over-the-counter orthotics. Dr. Pilar Almy, a Seattle-area podiatrist, recommends visiting shoe specialty shops to buy orthotics, as opposed to purchasing them at your local pharmacy. At an athletics shop, an outdoor store, or a running gear shop, a clerk versed in your sport and footwear will have you try on several styles of shoes, watching your gait as you jump, hike, or run. Often stores will have treadmills so they can watch your gait while you run or walk. Besides guiding you to specific footwear, a clerk can point out suitable orthotics for your gait issues. Dr. Almy recommends the following brands to her patients:

- Superfeet
- Sole
- Biosoft
- Quick-Stride
- Lyncos

Even if you don't have pronation or supination issues during your everyday life, participating in athletics might exaggerate a minor gait defect. This is why getting fitted for your athletic shoes is a good idea.

Muscles That Matter

The muscles that help move and stabilize our spine are numerous. It's useful to know about a handful of these muscles and their roles in back health. First up: The *multifidus muscle* is an important spine stabilizer. This muscle connects each vertebra to the next while also spanning more than one vertebra at a time. Having a strong multifidus muscle helps keep your spine stable, preventing injury and helping you perform on any athletic field.

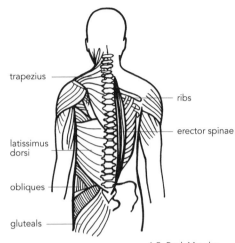

1.5. Back Muscles

Place your hands on either side of your spinal column; your *erector spinae muscles* lie along both sides of your backbone. These long muscles help keep the spine upright. The *gluteal muscles,* located in your buttocks, are usually some of the body's strongest muscles. These powerful muscles help you walk, run, and jump.

The much-discussed *abdominal muscles* have four layers, forming part of the core girdle. The so-called six-pack muscle is the *rectus abdominus;* this is the outer layer of the abdominal muscle. It helps us flex and prevents too much extension. Although people like to tout this muscle in public, the deeper abdominal muscles are even more valuable when it comes to building a strong lower back. Next up are the *external oblique muscles:* running from the rib cage to the pelvis, these muscles lend us rotational ability. The *internal oblique muscles* run at a 90-degree angle to the external oblique muscles. Together the external and internal oblique muscles form a cylinder of strength. The *transverse abdominus* is your fourth and deepest layer of abdominal muscles. Thought of as a primary spine stabilizer, this muscle surrounds the spine.

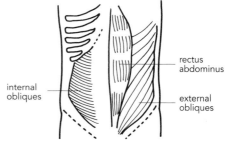

1.6. Abdominal Muscles

The next term on our list sounds magnificent and mysterious: *iliopsoas* (pronounced *"ill-eo-so-as"*). These muscles, which are also called hip flexor muscles, tie several body parts together. Iliopsoas muscles attach at the fronts of the lumbar vertebrae, cross over the pelvis, and insert onto the inside of the thigh as well as joining with muscles in the bowl of each side of your pelvis. These muscles link back movements to pelvis and thigh movements. If your iliopsoas muscles are tight, you might feel tension and possibly pain in your low back. How do these muscles get tight? Too much sitting is one culprit. Or perhaps you run fifty miles a week, but you rarely stretch these muscles.

Words You'll Hear Again

The preceding short list is by no means a complete picture of the muscles that support your lower back. Still, your physical therapist, yoga teacher, or Pilates instructor will probably mention these muscles in everyday conversations. You'll also hear talk of a *core girdle* and *training the core muscles*. Sometimes people believe just the abdominal muscles—and possibly the pelvic floor muscles—create this girdle. Actually, the core is a large rectangle of muscles extending from your knees all the way to your neck, supporting you on the front, back, and sides. Learning how to use these muscles with strength, endurance, power, and coordination is quite valuable. Without this muscle support system, our spines would collapse. Having a backbone without muscles is like hoping your tent poles will stay up without ropes and stakes.

Tendons and Ligaments

Muscles create motion with the help of *tendons*: Tendons usually connect muscles to bones, with a tendon at each end of every muscle. Tendons both help you move and hold your bones in place. *Ligaments* connect bone to bone. Three different ligaments run the length of the spine, connecting the vertebrae and helping to stop your spine from moving too far while you reach to catch that fly ball. The *anterior longitudinal ligament* attaches to the front of each vertebral body—that block of bone at the front of your vertebrae. The *posterior longitudinal ligament* attaches at the back of a vertebral body. The *supraspinous ligament* attaches at the tips of your spinous processes, those bony knobs you felt as you moved your fingertips along your backbone.

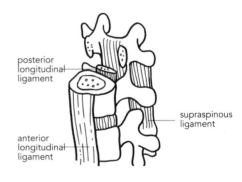

1.7. Ligaments

Both ligaments and tendons are composed of *collagen tissue,* which is usually round and very tough, similar in nature to leather. Both tendons and ligaments can stretch too far, resulting in injury.

2   THE MIND-BODY CONNECTION

WHEN YOUR BACK HURTS, it would be convenient if you could point to just one of the numerous parts and say, "There's the culprit. It's the facet joints on my L5 vertebra."

Unfortunately, low-back pain is not so simple. For starters, the back is a complex matrix, and every part with nerve endings—muscles, bones, facet joints, the outer portion of the disks, ligaments, tendons, and the nerves themselves—can feel pain. An additional complicating factor is that the spine is connected to the brain, another intricate body part.

Everyone experiences pain differently, depending on anatomy, genetic factors, past and current life experiences, and belief systems. Two people can have the same herniated disk show up on their X-rays, but only one of them will be in pain. For example, Chris and Dan experienced a similar acute back injury. Since the initial injury, Chris's pain has continued to reoccur three times a year; Dan, on the other hand, has never experienced another episode of low-back pain. In another tale, Stacy and Beth both suffer from the same acute back injury, but Stacy's pain resolved within six weeks while Beth's injury turned into daily, chronic pain.

In these stories, the person's emotions may make the difference between who visits the doctor repeatedly and who recovers quickly and continues to play soccer twice a week. Research supports this statement. One study published in the *Journal of General Internal Medicine* in 2008, for example, suggested that acute low-back pain patients with higher expectations for speedy recovery were likely to show more improvement.

Pain has a physical component, but it also derives from our emotions. We tell ourselves a "story" about why we have low-back pain. One part of that tale is from our rational mind, the other part is the emotional angle. In the midst of illness, we sometimes ignore the emotional side, or we tell ourselves we are stupid for having certain feelings. But thinking that way overlooks the powerful role emotions play in the story of pain.

Both the rational explanation and the emotional component are part of the *mind–body connection*; that is, how our minds and the emotions, thoughts, and feelings emanating from them affect our bodies. *Holistic healing* looks at the whole person, both the physical and emotional selves. It addresses not only the physical symptoms, but also the intellectual and emotional experiences associated with the pain.

WHAT EXACTLY HURTS?

"People think of pain as residing in the body, but it actually resides in your brain. This pain has some relationship to what is happening in your body, but it's not a one-to-one thing. If X happens in your body, then Y is not always happening in your brain. If that were the case, you would be able to figure out where the pain is coming from and why," explains Dr. Heather Kroll, a physiatrist and cofounder of the Rehabilitation Institute of Washington.

The body's sensory and pain-perceiving system is complicated. If you cut your finger, first you experience the feeling of the cut—a mild pain that doesn't hurt much. Over the next hours and days, the nervous system initiates an *inflammatory response* to start the healing process. Impulses sent to the brain trigger a response that sends chemicals to the injured area. These chemicals irritate the nerves around the cut, and then you feel more pain. Now that simple cut has sensitive, almost bruised, skin around it. You ask what hurts, and the answer is no longer simple.

Back pain is similar in nature. Perhaps you strain a ligament, which causes the muscles around that ligament to spasm. Then the muscles alter their normal movement, causing pain when you move in a certain way. Perhaps that alteration of movement also puts pressure on nearby joints, causing yet another source of pain.

When a body part hurts, it sends perception messages to the brain about what is happening to the injury, including tactile sensations, movement, temperature differences, and chemical and mechanical irritabilities.

In the brain, there is a map of our body, but it's a very distorted map. This map is primarily a guide to our skin, with large areas devoted to the fingers, mouth, and tongue, for example. Very tiny areas of this map are devoted to your back. There isn't a part of the brain that says, "This is the T12 vertebra." When you cut your finger, the brain map localizes that injury very well. When you strain a back muscle, however, that sensory experience is more diffuse: there is no pinpoint location on the map. Sensing an injury, the brain sends an inflammatory response to the back muscle, which causes spasms and other side effects to the injury, so now the pain encompasses more real estate.

The prevailing theory regarding *referred pain* adds another layer to this puzzle. When you pull a back muscle, the perception messages go to the brain on pain pathways. On these pain pathways, other structures that enter the spinal cord at that level can get stimulated. The "pain" experience is now happening to other parts of your body. For example, L4/L5 and S1/L5 disk pain can refer pain to the groin area. Likewise, some of the back's facet joints often refer pain to the lumbar spine, even though the pain started north of there.

DO EMOTIONS CREATE BACK PAIN?

If you discuss your sore back with your doctor, you may hear one of the following terms: *acute, subacute,* or *chronic.* An acute injury—whether you feel pain from a specific incident or it seemingly came out of nowhere—resolves itself within six weeks, leaving you pain free. Subacute pain persists past six weeks and up to three months. When you suffer from low-back pain for more than three months, it is called chronic pain. People with chronic pain usually experience pain every day.

What role do emotions play in the original onset of low-back pain symptoms? According to a systematic review of studies reported in a 1995 issue of *Spine,* symptoms of psychological distress in individuals without back pain predict the subsequent onset of new episodes of low-back pain. If Paul and Jim take similar tumbles on the basketball court, Paul's fall may result in a back injury while Jim doesn't suffer any consequences. Paul's work stresses and anxiety levels may have contributed to his back injury, while Jim's low level of emotional stress may have helped him avoid injury.

Once you have had one bout of low-back pain, it's common to have future episodes. You may have acute flare-ups of pain that come and go. Sometimes you can see a connection between these flare-ups and your activities; in other cases, a flare-up might not seem to have any logical connection to your actions. Emotions again may be an important factor in your recurring low-back pain, sometimes turning acute pain into chronic pain. A summary of studies reported in the *Journal of Occupational Rehabilitation* showed a strong association between psychological factors and future back pain. Job satisfaction, demands, stress, and perceived ability to work were related to back pain problems. A review of studies reported in *Spine* in 2002 showed that psychological factors such as stress and depressive mood might strongly influence the transition to chronic low-back pain.

Our mind has a role in all of these types of pain. How we experience the pain associated with acute, subacute, and chronic problems links to our emotions.

Your Life and Back Pain

Low-back pain can affect every aspect of your life. While psychosocial factors such as fear of pain, depression, and strained family relationships might cause acute pain to become chronic pain, sometimes the reverse can be true, with your low-back pain leading to psychosocial factors. For example, the life changes caused by your injury may leave you feeling depressed. Are you experiencing any of the following psychosocial factors?

- You avoid activities such as your twice-weekly run due to fear of pain.
- You expect your pain to increase during your workday or while you push your toddler's stroller on your daily walk.
- You focus excessively on your pain, talking about it with everyone you meet or thinking about it for major portions of your day.
- You suffer from feelings of helplessness.
- You feel depressed, irritable, and/or anxious.
- You have trouble falling asleep or staying asleep.

THE STORY OF PAIN

Every low-back pain has a story. "Like all experiences, pain is influenced by everything that is going on in a person's life at the time, and probably by everything that has gone on in the past," says Dr. J. David Sinclair, pain management specialist in Seattle. "Pain, when considered as an experience, offers many more useful therapeutic options than the idea that pain is a thing that can be killed with pain-killers or cut out with surgery to remove the so-called pain generator."

If the pain resolves quickly, we don't always connect the story to our emotions. Maybe we talk about physical causes, saying, "I think carrying my toddler around resulted in a lumbar spine strain," or "My forty-year-old back gave out on the racquetball court." That might be just part of the story: emotions may have predisposed you to getting this acute injury.

The stories we tell ourselves are not only part of developing acute pain, but also play a role in reoccurrences of back pain and the

Other psychosocial factors stem from our personal histories, including a history of substance, physical, or sexual abuse, or a background of other disabling injuries and conditions. Studies show psychosocial issues, often called "yellow flags" by physicians, are the primary precursors of a patient's acute pain becoming chronic pain. A study published by the international journal *Spine* in 1991 followed more than three thousand employees at the Boeing Aircraft Company. Three hundred workers suffered from disabling development of chronic pain. For example, if we get an acute back injury, we might recall that our favorite aunt hurt her back and ended up in a wheelchair. We might start imagining ourselves unable to work. These tales cause our back pain to intensify. Stress, fear, and anger can make muscles tense up. We worry that the low-back pain will never go away. We recall that Uncle Jim stopped playing sports due to his bad back. Although acute and sub-acute pain often resolve within three months, the emotions tied to these injuries can help lead to chronic pain.

One tool that can help change the story we tell ourselves about pain is meditation. Through daily meditation, we can deal with the emotional stressors that help intensify pain. For more information, turn to Chapter 6, "Practices for the Mind."

back pain during the four-year timeframe. The top predictor of disabling low-back pain was emotional stress from a person's job. Stress from psychological issues was also a better indicator of disabling back problems than physical issues, such as sitting all day or lifting heavy objects.

Similar in nature to psychosocial factors is the idea that your pain is taking place in a context. The layers of experience that surround chronic back problems are different for every person, but many doctors feel addressing the contextual issues can help people both manage and ease their pain. Any issue that can magnify a person's stress can help contribute to pain and is worth examining.

For example, it's helpful for a practitioner to know your cultural beliefs. If you believe a person in pain should rest in bed for one year while his family cares for him, this is vital information. Layers of context can include, but are not limited to, the following factors:

- Relationships with spouses, children, parents, relatives, coworkers, and friends
- Work, whether that means your current stressful work situation or the fact that you no longer work due to disabling back pain
- Medicine: are the current prescriptions working well?
- Childhood issues, from something as simple as how you learned to deal with pain to complex issues such as physical and sexual abuse
- Current home environment and its stressors
- Daily activities, including both the activities you have trouble doing every day and the physical and social activities in which you have stopped participating
- Depression, anxiety, or sleep problems

These layers can add stress and conflict to a person's life, which intensify the severity of pain. Addressing the whole person can have a very real, positive effect on a person with low-back pain.

The Fight-or-Flight Response

The psychosocial factors associated with pain as well as current life stressors can be understood in terms of a common fifth-grade social studies lesson. The fight-or-flight response lesson we learned as children often involved a tiger or a lion and went something like this: Picture yourself in a jungle. You are going about your everyday duties, collecting drinking water from a small pond. Suddenly you feel a set of eyes looking at you. You spy a tiger in a nearby tree. This threat causes a physical response in your body: your heart pounds loud and fast, you sweat, and all your muscles tense as your body prepares for action.

This acute stress response is vital in your jungle situation. You either fight the tiger or flee as fast as your feet will carry you. In some modern-day scenarios, this stress response is also helpful, such as when you encounter a threatening stranger on a dark city street. Still, this heightened arousal can be harmful in other situations. Perhaps we don't have a full throttle fight-or-flight response when something goes awry, but even a lower stress response can cause tension in the body. Parenting issues, a confrontation with a boss, or dealing with your divorce can create some level of tension in the mind and body. Add a back injury to this equation, and suddenly the heightened mind–body arousal makes the back pain worse.

The stress created in our minds can cause the muscle tension in our bodies to increase. This stress can be from all kinds of emotions, such as anger, fear, and anxiety. If we have too much stress in our lives, or if we are not dealing well with stress, this muscle tension can become constant. Some practitioners believe this ever-present muscle tension transforms acute low-back pain into a chronic condition.

TENSION MYOSITIS SYNDROME

We've talked about the emotional component of illness: how pain can cause an emotional reaction in the body. We've discussed how emotions affect the body: how stress can help worsen pain. A physician named John Sarno takes the mind–body connection a step further. In his 1981 book, *Mind Over Back Pain,* Sarno introduced a condition called *Tension Myositis Syndrome,* or TMS. Sarno postulates that back pain and other manifestations of pain are most often brought on by myofascial or muscle/tissue pain. The pain can manifest in numerous ways: tinnitus, repetitive stress syndrome, headache, irritable bowel syndrome, and so forth. Most importantly, repressed emotions— usually anger or rage—initially cause the muscle tension and pain. With TMS, repressed emotional stress is the root of the back pain. TMS has nothing to do with readily expressed and processed emotions. Instead, TMS is about repressed emotions buried deep inside a chronic pain patient.

There are very few TMS practitioners; perhaps fewer than twenty doctors in the United States are versed in dealing with TMS. Some people with low-back pain read Sarno's books and treat themselves. Mark G. Strom, MD, a medical acupuncturist and integrative heath physician in Seattle, is a TMS practitioner. Dr. Strom, a retired cardiac surgeon, believes a TMS practitioner is a person to see alongside your primary care provider after a medical work-up has produced insufficient relief. When Dr. Strom sees a new patient, he reviews medical records, takes a complete medical history, and completes a physical exam. The TMS treatment is similar to psychological therapy, but doesn't follow the confines of traditional therapies. Dr. Strom feels the intimate rapport built between the patient and the TMS practitioner is the defining characteristic of his practice's success. He creates a safe space for patients that creates a wall of confidentiality and is available 24/7, allowing the patient to face and deal with whatever emotions are leading to the pain.

Often, the patients Dr. Strom sees have tried and had little success with numerous other options, both medical and surgical, to relieve their chronic pain. Sometimes the patients are skeptical that repressed emotions could cause their pain. But if they feel better, it doesn't matter which came first, the emotions or the physical hurt.

The Chronic-Pain Cycle

Stress—along with other emotions—feeds into a chronic-pain cycle. Let's say you start with a pulled muscle in your lumbar spine. First, you experience pain from the strain. Then the stress from your everyday life adds more muscle tension to the injury site, creating more hurt. You notice that roughhousing with your kids really makes your back hurt. Now you fear this daily playtime and you avoid this activity. Thoughts of your father come to mind: he didn't play sports because of his bad back.

All of these psychological factors lead you to restrict your own physical activities. Your muscles become deconditioned due to lack of use. Soon enough, your flexibility, endurance, and strength are affected. Perhaps your emotions start playing a larger role: You are frustrated that you can't play with your kids, angry that your injury has changed your life, and fearful of undertaking what used to be normal movements for your body. Now you avoid engaging in activities that you used to enjoy.

Both the psychological and physical factors are part of the chronic-pain cycle. This cycle creates more hurt and makes healing much more difficult.

Preventing a "Chronic-Pain Identity"

Sometimes your life becomes all about your back pain. When we have pain, especially chronic pain, we can easily become emotionally distressed. This makes the pain worse. When the pain gets worse, this triggers more emotional distress, and this actually triggers more pain. You are stuck like a gerbil in a wheel, wondering what happened to your old, vibrant self. Your daily existence may not resemble what it looked like before back pain took center stage. But this doesn't have to happen. There are two primary ways to avoid letting chronic back pain take over your life.

First, you must deal with the loss. If you have forever lost certain abilities, you need to grieve that loss. This is similar to grieving the loss of a loved one. In the process, you may experience denial, depression, anger, bargaining, and acceptance at various times, and not necessarily in that order. A therapist versed in pain management can help with this process.

The other key component is to focus on the positive and what you can do to empower yourself. Remember the things you loved about your old life. Perhaps, before you started suffering from low-back pain, you used to practice martial arts. You stopped because you thought the pain would make it impossible to continue that activity. On the contrary, tapping back in to those martial art skills—from the breathing techniques to using the muscular training in your current daily exercises—can help you deal with your pain. You can set a goal to participate in martial arts again. Instead of believing that you no longer can engage in activities you once loved, you have to change your mind set to realize that getting back into martial arts or rejoining your hiking club might be possible.

Both of the above processes will help you understand that you have a life outside the experience of pain. You can still participate in many activities and have a happy existence, even while experiencing bouts of low-back hurt. Perhaps it is a different life, but it still has merit and good times.

Hope

Sometimes a person suffering from chronic low-back pain thinks he cannot get better. He lacks hope. Perhaps this is because he has been in pain for years. Maybe it is because his practitioners don't appear optimistic about his situation. Whatever the reason, the lack of hope can perpetuate the problem. Hope is often a necessary ingredient in relieving pain.

THE GLASS IS EMPTY

Sometimes, mental health counseling can be helpful for people with chronic low-back pain. Think about seeking psychological counseling if stress, fear, anxiety, and similar emotions start to affect your perception of the pain, and the hurt takes center stage in your life. If you are suffering from depression or anxiety, or if you see yourself as trapped in a tunnel of pain, undergoing psychological counseling can be imperative. Look for a counselor who has worked with chronic-pain patients. Therapists without pain management experience may not know the best avenues for easing suffering.

Often professionals who specialize in therapy for chronic-pain sufferers are cognitive or cognitive behavioral therapists. Cognitive therapists try to challenge the distorted or negative thoughts a patient can be thinking; these thoughts can help keep the patient in a chronic-pain cycle. A cognitive behavioral therapist also works to change the behaviors that may be impairing the patient.

A patient and counselor need to establish a caring, trusting relationship. "The relationship is the treatment," says Dr. Alan Weisser, a pain management psychologist at Seattle-based New Options. He sees his role as showing patients that they already have the tools to help make themselves better.

A person suffering from chronic low-back pain may not realize self-deprecating thoughts can add to his pain and keep him from enjoying his life. In therapy, patients work to understand how their emotions, thought patterns, moods, and stressors contribute to chronic low-back pain. Patients also create coping strategies that alleviate stressors.

If you suffer from depression, a therapist might prescribe antidepressant medication. Whether or not these medications are nec-essary, you will be encouraged to re-engage in daily activities, such as exercise, social activities, and household chores. This counteracts depression and shows people they can experience pain while still participating fully in their lives.

In *The Anatomy of Hope: How People Prevail in the Face of Illness*, Dr. Jerome Groopman writes that belief and expectation are the defining elements of hope. One of the reasons people need hope is scientific, writes Groopman:

Belief and expectation ... can block pain by releasing the brain's endorphins and enkephalins, mimicking the effects of morphine. In some cases, hope can also have important effects on fundamental physiological processes like respiration, circulation, and motor function. During the course of an illness, then, hope can be imagined as a domino effect, a chain reaction in which each link makes improvement more likely. It changes us profoundly in spirit and in body.

Believing and expecting that you will feel better helps move you forward, completing physical tasks and feeling positive about the future. If you feel hopeless about your back pain, getting better most likely is out of your grasp. This doesn't mean you need to find a practitioner who promises a cure. Chronic pain is most often about management, not a 100 percent cure. Believing you can feel better, as well as believing you can have a productive, happy life despite the pain, is valuable. Hope needs to be steeped in reality, but the inspiration and support it offers can make a critical difference in how you live your life.

3 COMMON BACK PROBLEMS

LOW-BACK PAIN IS NOT A NEW PHENOMENON. Literary back pain references date back thousands of years. The earliest known instance might be in Egyptian surgical papyrus papers from the seventeenth century BC discovered by Edwin Smith. Hippocrates, considered the father of medicine, wrote about back pain. In the Bible, Esau's angel touched Jacob on the hip during a wrestling match. Afterwards, Jacob walked with a limp.

In today's terms, Jacob suffered from sciatica. According to Jewish law, butchers must dissect the sciatic nerve in the hindquarters of beef to make it kosher.

Still, the first back surgery did not occur until 1934. Spine specialist Dr. Stan Herring, who practices at the University of Washington in Seattle, believes the disability associated with back pain is recent. "Since time immemorial, there's been low-back pain, but I don't remember reading about legions of Roman soldiers on disability," says Herring.

Back pain has become a big part of the medical industry. While this means researchers are looking for solutions, it also means that people tend to think of low-back pain as a disease. This leads people on the hunt for one cure, instead of thinking of this hurt as a more normal occurrence. Looking for a quick remedy can cause anxiety and stress.

It's not that people shouldn't seek ways to alleviate pain, but it is helpful to shine a different light on lumbar spine issues. For example, a 1997 public health campaign in Australia illuminated the fact that low-back pain is typically not a serious medical problem. The campaign erected billboards and produced radio and television spots with messages such as, "Does your back hurt? Get up and take a walk," and "Back pain—don't take it lying down." The campaign conveyed that engaging in the daily activities of life is often the best treatment for low-back pain. During and directly after the campaign, the rate of medical payments for back claims fell by more than 25 percent.

People can avoid undue worry by seeing low-back pain as a part of life. As we age, degenerative changes make low-back pain a real possibility for almost all of us. But we'll all get wrinkles, too. As you peruse the following descriptions of back problems, think of low-back pain as a condition, not a disease.

SEEKING A DIAGNOSIS

If you have back pain, you're not alone. At this moment, 31 million people in the United States experience symptoms of lumbar spine pain. If your back hurts right now, it would be great to know exactly why you are in pain. Is the injury from too much trail-running over boulder-strewn paths?

The good news: running most likely didn't cause your problem, even if the injury occurred while you were jogging down a mountain trail. The misstep that left you in agony was the final trigger point. Most likely, your low back has been getting weaker for a while now. Think about the twinges of pain leading up to this moment, while you were sitting in an uncomfortable working position or as you reached for the box of camping supplies in the garage.

The bad news: your problem probably doesn't have a specific diagnosis. The most common diagnosis for lumbar back pain is "nonspecific low-back pain." If you visit your doctor for your injury, 85 percent of the time she'll tell you, "I don't know what exactly is wrong with you."

This great mystery is due to all the mind–body factors discussed in Chapter 2, and it boils down to this: the back is a complex structure with many different parts that can feel pain. Weave in the fact that the spine connects to the brain, adding another layer of complexity. The body's sensory and pain-perceiving systems are not simple.

Still, don't worry if your doctor is unable to give you a pinpoint diagnosis for your low-back pain. If you are not hurting in a way that is quite worrisome, it doesn't usually matter which body part is the instigator of the pain. Nonspecific back pain is treatable, and your hurt can still be relieved.

RED FLAGS

When low-back pain flares up, it's important to be aware of possible "red flag" symptoms. These are warning signs that should alert you to possible serious problems associated with low-back pain. In fact, when you do visit a care provider, her first responsibility is make sure you have no red flag symptoms, ruling out the possibility of medical conditions that need immediate treatment.

If you are experiencing lumbar spine pain along with any of the following symptoms, see your doctor as soon as possible:

- Unexplained weight loss
- Resting or night pain
- Fever
- Recent infection
- Urinary retention
- Fecal incontinence
- Loss of sensation in buttocks and perineum
- Recent trauma
- Abdominal pulsating mass
- Significant weakness
- Progressive muscle weakness

Risk Factors

Some risk factors are often associated with more serious low-back pain issues. Your doctor will need this information during your appointment. Be sure to visit your physician if you have lumbar spine pain and one or more of the following risk factors:

- History of cancer
- History of osteoporosis
- Use of corticosteroids and immune-suppressing drugs
- Age greater than fifty years
- Intravenous drug use
- Pain lasting longer than six weeks

SPASMS, STRAINS, AND SPRAINS

Symptoms: If you are experiencing pain, tightness, spasms, or tender muscles in your lower back, you are probably suffering from a *muscle soft-tissue injury*. This is also called a *lumbar strain* or *sprain*, or even a *sprain-strain injury*. Sometimes you'll feel worse when you are bending forward or to the side. Also, your lower back might be stiff and more painful in the morning, feeling better as you move through the day. You may not be able to point to one specific locale as the pain source, since the hurt may radiate into various areas of your body. For example, your low-back pain and tenderness may extend into your buttocks.

Explanation: Lumbar sprain-strain or muscle soft-tissue injury is also called *myofascial pain*, which simply means muscle (*myo*) tissue (*fascia*) pain. The hurt stems from injury to muscles, ligaments, tendons, connective tissue, joints, or cartilage in the back. A strain-sprain happens when the fibers of ligaments, tendons, or muscles tear a tiny bit or are pulled out of their natural alignment. A spasm occurs when a body part becomes strained and then the pain of the injury causes the nervous system to send out signals for the muscles to actively contract. These painful muscle spasms might keep you from moving, hindering the healing process. Sometimes the fibers of ligaments or muscles actually tear in response to trauma, an injury, or a fall. If you tear these fibers—now your injury is called a *muscle tear*—you are going to know it happened: it will be a traumatic event.

Causes: Bad posture or being in poor physical shape can lead to lumbar strains. Sometimes this injury is associated with an actual event, such as lifting a heavy object, improperly moving an item, sleeping in an awkward position, or repeating a certain motion. Usually this event is the trigger point in a cascade of events leading up to the actual injury. Your low-back pain might have been developing for years. You might recall twinges of pain the last time you went backpacking, for example. If the final event—a collision on the soccer field—leads to the injury, this doesn't mean you need to avoid playing soccer once you heal from this episode of pain. You might need to pay more attention to the way you move on any athletic field, though.

A sprain-strain injury usually happens during everyday activities. Something as simple as landing wrong while running or reaching to put a glass away in the cupboard can precede this injury. Of course, the action that leads to the hurt can be more dramatic—overexerting yourself on a weeklong backpacking trip or twisting too much to make that shot on the squash court. The physical changes brought on by pregnancy can also lead to lumbar strains and sprains.

Treatment: The good news is that spasms, strains, and sprains usually heal quite easily. Typically, muscle soft-tissue injuries resolve within six weeks time. The best treatment for these back problems is relative rest. For one to three days, avoid tasks that cause too much pain. ("Relative rest," however, doesn't mean going to bed for two days or parking yourself in your favorite recliner. You need to keep moving to heal faster.) People tend to guard and protect their low back when it hurts, altering the way they move. The less time you spend in this guarded movement pattern, the better. Resume normal activities and movement patterns as soon as possible; this is the key to healing.

You can ice your lower back for the first seventy-two hours. Icing may help ease pain and decrease local swelling. If applying heat helps you feel better, you can do this after seventy-two hours. (See the box "Ice or Heat?" below.) Take over-the-counter (OTC) pain relief medications such as aspirin, ibuprofen, Tylenol, or topical analgesic creams. These medications alleviate pain and swelling, which can help you get your back moving as quickly as possible. Although there are side effects for OTC medications, usually these side effects occur while using OTC medications for an extended period. (For more information on pain medications, see Chapter 9.)

A holistic approach is ideal for treating low-back strains, sprains, and spasms. Later chapters in this book discuss various therapies and practices that can be immensely helpful in addressing low-back pain. Remember the spokes on the wheel—the variety of therapies from which you can choose? Consider any of the following, alone or in combination:

- A bodyworks practitioner, such as a massage therapist, an acupuncturist, or a chiropractor, can ease your pain and offer symptom relief (see Chapter 7).
- Practicing meditation may help lessen the hurt (see Chapter 6).
- Yoga, Pilates, and tai chi are movement therapies that can both relieve pain and possibly prevent pain and future strains or sprains (see Chapter 5).
- You can also ease painful inflammation by changing your diet (see Chapter 8).

If you are unable to get moving after three days, visit your primary care physician or a physiatrist (a doctor trained in physical medicine and rehabilitation). Your doctor can prescribe medications to ease pain, allowing you to resume the activities of daily life.

ICE OR HEAT?

Heat or cold packs can help relieve back pain. After you injure your lumbar spine, use ice for the first seventy-two hours. Then, if warmth feels better to you, switch to a heat pack. A cold pack eases inflammation and decreases muscle spasms, while heat packs enhance blood flow. Sometimes people alternate cold and heat. Place heat or ice packs on your injury for approximately twenty minutes at a time, every few hours.

If you have been in pain for a while now, or you are suffering from chronic pain, rate your pain on a scale of zero to ten, with ten being the worst pain. If your back pain is a three in the morning, but grows to a six in the evening, this is most likely a sign of inflammation. Treat your pain with an ice pack. If your pain stays a steady three throughout the day and night, use a heat pack.

Ice packs can take several forms. Try a bag of frozen vegetables, such as peas or corn. Buy ice packs at your local drugstore or just put some ice cubes in a Ziploc baggie. Don't let ice touch your sensitive skin; place a thin towel between the ice and your low back.

Heat options include heating pads, moist heating pads, or even warming up a slightly damp hand towel in your microwave. Over-the-counter Thermacare heat packs also can increase blood flow. These can alleviate pain during long car rides or airplane trips, during athletic activities, or while sleeping.

Since we are speaking of slumbering, try resting on your side in a fetal position. Placing a pillow between your legs can also relieve pain. Back sleepers can put a pillow or rolled towels beneath their knees.

DISK TEARS, DISK BULGES, AND HERNIATED DISKS

Symptoms: *Disk tears, bulges,* and *herniations* might not hurt. Often a person suffering from back pain will have an MRI image taken of his back. A disk herniation will appear on the film, leading to a diagnosis of the disk herniation being the cause of the pain. This seems perfectly apt, unless you consider several studies that look at back MRIs of the general population. A study by Maureen C. Jensen of Harvard and reported in *The New England Journal of Medicine* in 1994 showed that 30 percent of the people who had abnormal disks experienced no pain. Some doctors quote studies that put the number of people with disk abnormalities who are not feeling any pain associated with the herniations at all at a full 50 percent. As with other types of low-back pain, you may have had an abnormal disk for years before you started experiencing pain, and the current hurt might or might not be from that abnormal disk. If you do have pain from a lumbar spine disk injury, the hurt might feel similar to lumbar strain symptoms. Symptoms can include pain tightness, tenderness, or spasms in your low back. Other symptoms stemming from disk herniations include sharp, stabbing, shooting, or burning pain. A disk bulge or tear can also irritate, pinch, or compress a nerve root or roots (see the "Pinched Nerves" section later in this chapter).

Explanation: By the age of thirty, the disks between our vertebrae can begin to degenerate. They lose water content and can shrink in height, which provides less space and cushioning between the bones of our spine. As a disk starts to degenerate, a disk tear, bulge, or herniation is more likely to happen. Picture the soft center of the disk, called the *nucleus pulposus*, as a water balloon, and the *annulus fibrosis* as the ring around that balloon. As

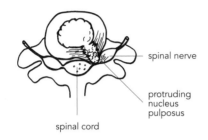

spinal nerve

protruding nucleus pulposus

spinal cord

3.1. Disk Herniation

we get older, we can get microscopic tears in that ring. Eventually, the nucleus pulposus can protrude out into one of these tears, resulting in a disk bulge or protrusion. A disk herniation occurs when a sudden increase in the tearing of the outer ring causes the inner nucleus pulposus to actually break through the outer ring. The soft center material now makes its way outside the disk. Most disk herniations occur between the L4 and L5 vertebrae and the L5 and S1 vertebrae. Other terms for disk herniation include *prolapsed disk* or *slipped disk*.

Causes: No traumatic event is necessary for a disk tear or bulge to take place; something as simple as tying your shoe can activate this hurt. If you are over the age of thirty, a disk herniation can happen in the course of everyday life. If you are younger, it usually takes a significant injury, such as a car accident, a fall while horseback riding, or a skateboarding crash, to produce a disk bulge, tear, or herniation. Of course, even after the age of thirty, a traumatic event can cause a disk herniation: lifting a forty-pound backpack while you are in a less-than-ideal posture, a car accident, or falling while skiing. The effects of pregnancy on a body can cause disk bulge or herniation. Still, it is remarkably uncommon to have one event cause a disk herniation. Several events over a lifetime often lead to this injury, starting with the back pain you felt after a gymnastic injury in high school. Add in degenerative changes that happen as you age or a genetic predisposition to back injuries, and eventually you injure one or more disks in your low back. Risk factors for disk herniation also include obesity and repeated heavy lifting.

Treatment: As with muscle soft-tissue injury, the first step in caring for disk bulges and herniations is pain relief. Easing your pain allows you to resume normal activities as soon as possible. For the first few days after a disk injury, get relative rest: avoid activities that cause your back to hurt, but try to be as active as possible. Once again, moving your body leads to healing.

Ice your low back for the first seventy-two hours; after that, you can use heat or ice to ease pain (see the box "Ice or Heat?" in this chapter). Take OTC pain relief medications such as aspirin, ibuprofen, and topical analgesic creams. See Chapter 6 to learn how meditation and hypnotherapy can lessen pain and Chapter 8 to learn how changing your diet can lessen inflammation.

If these treatments fail to ease your hurt, book an appointment with your primary care physician. She can prescribe prescription medications. Your doctor also might recommend seeing a physiatrist (nerve, muscle, and bone expert trained in physical medicine and rehabilitation), a physical therapist, a massage therapist, or a chiropractor. If she doesn't suggest any of these therapies, ask her if you can try one of them to relieve pain and promote healing. (See Chapter 5 about finding movement professionals such as physiatrists, physical therapists, or instructors in yoga, Pilates, the Feldenkrais Method, or the Alexander Technique. See Chapter 7 for information about massage, chiropractic care, acupuncture, and other bodyworks therapies.)

If you don't improve, your doctor might recommend cortisone or epidural injections to ease swelling and pain. Sometimes doctors prescribe injections so you can lower your level of prescription medications (see Chapter 9 for more information on injections). You may have heard that disk herniations require surgery. This is a misconception: several studies show that after two years, people who have had surgery and people who have not had surgery recovered at equivalent rates (see the studies described in Chapter 9). Disk herniations that compress a nerve root or roots, causing severe or progressive leg pain, tingling, weakness, or numbness, might require surgery. (Read the "Pinched Nerves" section below, for more information.)

PINCHED NERVES

Symptoms: If you have an *irritated, pinched,* or *compressed nerve root,* you might feel pain that radiates or shoots out from an area in your low back, spreading to your buttocks and sometimes radiating into one or both legs and feet. This pain is traveling along a nerve root pathway. You also might feel weakness, tingling, numbness, or loss of reflexes in one or both legs and feet.

Symptoms of weakness, tingling, numbness, and loss of reflexes, especially if severe or affecting the bowel, bladder, or groin, could also be from a rare condition called *cauda equina syndrome.* Permanent nerve damage can result from cauda equina syndrome. Therefore, if you experience any of the symptoms listed above, see a doctor immediately to rule out cauda equina syndrome and other red flag concerns (if your doctor is unavailable, go to the ER).

Explanation: The nerve roots in your back branch off the spinal cord, exiting the canal through gaps in the spinal canal called *foramen*. A pinched nerve means a nerve root or roots are irritated, impinged upon, or compressed. This is also called *radicular pain* or *radiculopathy*. This impingement can be mechanical in nature, from physical compression on the nerve or its blood supply, or it can be chemical, due to the inflammatory response set in motion by a disk herniation. Nerve impingement can cause tingling, numbness, loss of reflexes, or weakening in one leg and foot. If your sciatic nerve specifically is irritated or pinched, this is called *sciatic nerve pain*. (See the "Sciatic Nerve Pain" section later in this chapter.)

Causes: The inflammatory response from a disk herniation can cause nerve root irritation. A disk herniation can physically pinch or compress a nerve. Osteoarthritis, facet joint syndrome, spondylolisthesis, or degenerative disk disease can also cause nerve root irritation or compression.

Treatment: Self-care methods of pain relief include ice and heat therapy (see the box "Ice or Heat?" above), taking OTC pain-relief medications, and exercising within the parameters set by your doctor. Your primary care provider might prescribe either OTC or prescription pain-relief medication and will help you create a treatment plan. If a disk or other back part is impinging on a nerve root, medication is necessary to reduce the swelling and inflammation that is pinching the root. Your doctor might prescribe an epidural steroid injection (see Chapter 9 for information about injections). This might relieve your pain so you can participate in your daily life and start moving your body again.

Depending on where you are in your healing process, your doctor might recommend one or more complementary treatments. See later chapters in this book for information about such treatments. They include the following:

- A bodyworks practitioner, such as a massage therapist, an acupuncturist, or a chiropractor, can ease your pain and offer symptom relief (see Chapter 7).
- Yoga, Pilates, and tai chi are movement therapies that can both relieve pain and possibly prevent pain and future injuries (see Chapter 5).
- Practicing meditation might help lessen the hurt (see Chapter 6).
- You can also ease painful inflammation by changing your diet (see Chapter 8).

Sometimes surgery is necessary if a disk herniation is physically impinging on a nerve root, causing severe and progressive pain, weakness, tingling, or numbness. If you only have back pain from a pinched nerve, surgery is not likely to relieve your pain. If you have both back *and* leg pain, surgery may be successful at relieving leg pain, although it may or may not ease your back pain. Refer to Chapter 9 for a thorough discussion about the pros and cons of back surgery.

OSTEOARTHRITIS

Symptoms: If you are under the age of thirty, you are unlikely to experience symptoms of osteoarthritis; if you are over the age of sixty, you are much more prone to suffering such symptoms. Often you will feel a localized pain, stemming from inflammation, in and around the arthritic facet joint or joints. Usually you'll feel more pain and have more swelling while you are actively moving; this pain and inflammation will fade while you are resting. You may feel stiff in the morning or after rest periods. You might not be able to move your back as freely as usual; the technical term for this is *limited range of motion.* Sometimes people hear a crackling sound as they move the affected joint or joints. Osteoarthritis might affect a nearby nerve root pathway, in which case you might have *referred pain,* meaning the pain is located far from the joint.

This disease does have one thing in common with herniated disks: two people can have MRI films that show similar amounts of osteoarthritis in their facet joints, but only one of them will experience pain. You and your care provider will want to explore whether the hurt stems from that arthritic facet joint or from something else entirely.

Explanation: Osteoarthritis is the most common form of arthritis. In your low back, osteoarthritis affects the facet joints of the spinal column. Remember, from Chapter 1, the four facet joints that jut out like arms and legs off the back of each vertebra, roughly resembling a headless stick-figure person? Smooth cartilage covers the surface of our facet joints. This connective tissue starts to degenerate with age, becoming thinner, with small tears in its surface. Because of the damage, bony growths called *osteophytes* can form. Osteoarthritis often causes an inflammatory response in the facet joints, leading to swelling and pain. The following factors can speed up this normal wear and tear on the facet joints: being overweight, having an injury or infection in the area, or suffering from congenital defects.

Extensive osteoarthritis of your facet joints can compress the nerves and the central canal that the spinal cord goes through. If this occurs in the lumbar spine, it is called *lumbar stenosis. Spinal stenosis* can occur for other reasons, including genetics (for more information, see the "Spinal Stenosis" section below).

Causes: Often defined as *wear-and-tear arthritis*, osteoarthritis happens as people age. Although prior injuries and a family history of the disease are risk factors, everyone has some normal wear and tear on their joints as they get older.

Treatment: There are numerous forms of self-treatment for osteoarthritis. See other chapters in this book for information about such treatments. They include the following:

- You can use ice to ease inflammation (see the box "Ice or Heat?" above), and take OTC pain relief medications to ease swelling and pain (see Chapter 9).
- Simple aerobic exercise can diminish pain, as can movement therapies such as yoga, Pilates, tai chi, the Alexander Technique, and the Feldenkrais Method. Such therapies not only can help you move your body in ways that are less hurtful, but can also ease painful inflammation. (See Chapters 4 and 5 for information about these exercises and therapies.)
- Practicing meditation or hypnotherapy can be effective pain-relief options (see Chapter 6).
- Various forms of massage therapy, acupuncture, and chiropractic care might be helpful as well; turn to Chapter 7 for information on these practices.
- You also can alter your diet to lessen inflammation; see Chapter 8 for more information.

If you are unable to ease your pain, schedule an appointment with your primary care provider or a physiatrist. She might recommend injecting your facet joint with a steroid (see Chapter 9 for information about injections).

If steroid injections don't relieve your pain, your doctor might talk to you about Intradiscal Electrothermal Therapy (IDET), or facet rhizotomy. These procedures heat up the facet joint's nerve roots, which might stop the nerve root from sending pain messages to the brain.

DEGENERATIVE DISK DISEASE

Symptoms: The main symptom of degenerative disk disease is low-back pain. It can feel similar to a lumbar strain, with tightness and a restricted range of motion in your low back. Perhaps your low back hurts if you extend it too far—say reaching to catch a Frisbee toss. You might feel stiff in the morning or after resting. Often, however, people with degenerative disk disease have no symptoms at all, and this spinal problem is an incidental finding on an MRI or CT scan.

Explanation: As we age, our disks gradually lose their water content, shrinking in height, and providing less cushioning and space between the vertebrae. This is normal wear and tear. As with osteoarthritis and herniated disks, this degeneration causes pain in some people, while other people don't hurt at all. Although the word *disease* is in the title, a degenerative disk problem is akin to getting wrinkles. We all get wrinkles; hopefully, we don't think of wrinkles as a disease.

Because of shortened disk height, the space where our nerves exit the spinal canal—called the *foramen*—might narrow. Usually a combination of osteoarthritis and degenerative disk disease can cause the nerves exiting the narrowed spinal canal to become irritated or compressed. This same combination of diseases can also cause your facet joints—those backbone joints that ease movement and connect the vertebrae—to become misaligned.

Causes: Degenerative disk disease is part of the normal aging process. Everyone eventually has some degeneration in his or her disks, thanks to the glorious process of getting older.

Treatment: Usually you can treat degenerative disk disease by yourself. Refer to other chapters in this book to learn about self-treatment therapies, including the following:

- You can ease pain and inflammation with OTC pain relief medications; see Chapter 9 for information about such medications.
- Regular aerobic exercise can lessen pain. If you find moving or exercising painful, try a movement therapy. To expand your range of motion and prevent pain, stretch and strengthen your low back and its surrounding muscles. It's a good idea to exercise on a regular basis, as well. See Chapter 4 for information about stretches and exercises that can help.
- For pain relief, try practicing meditation (see Chapter 6).
- Seek help from a professional: physical therapy, various forms of massage therapy, acupuncture, hypnotherapy, and chiropractic care might be helpful (see Chapters 5 and 7).
- To learn how to ease inflammation through diet changes, turn to Chapter 8.

CRACKED OR SLIPPING VERTEBRAE

Symptoms: Like many back problems, a *cracked* or *slipping vertebra* might exist but exhibit no symptoms. If you play sports with lots of hyperextension—think gymnastics here—you might have back pain for two weeks or more. Even if you don't participate in athletics that put pressure on your low back, symptoms can include aching in your low back and tenderness

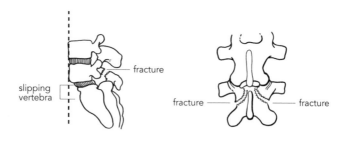

3.2. Spondylolisthesis

with bending, pain in the thighs and legs, muscle spasms, and tight or painful hamstring muscles. Neurologic symptoms are also possible: pain, weakness, tingling, or numbness in the low back, buttocks, leg or legs, and foot or feet.

Explanation: A cracked or fractured vertebra is called *spondylolysis*. This crack runs through the back part of the vertebral body, between the facet joints where the pedicles and lamina come together. (See fig. 1.2. for an illustration of the vertebra.) Spondylolysis can progress to *spondylolisthesis*, which is a slipping vertebra. Spondylolisthesis occurs when one vertebra slides forward or backward relative to another vertebra. This misalignment is labeled by degrees, going from a mild 1 to a severe 4. Sometimes a slipped disk can irritate or compress a nerve root or roots, leading to the neurological symptoms discussed above.

Causes: Spondylolysis often shows up in young athletes participating in sports with hyperextension, including gymnastics, ballet, and football.

Often spondylolysis isn't diagnosed until a person is older, although she might have experienced back problems as a teenager. Spondylolysis and spondylolisthesis can be present because the area never fused congenitally. This fracture can also occur later in life, sometimes from sports participation, but also from other causes such as degenerative changes in the vertebrae. Sports with lots of back extension are more likely to cause a cracked vertebra. Some sports, such as weight lifting and football, also put a lot of pressure on the low back.

Spondylolisthesis, or a slipped vertebra, can be the result of a cracked vertebra. Often people have a genetic predisposition toward spondylolisthesis. Degenerative changes in disks can also cause vertebrae to move out of alignment. As a disk loses its height, the vertebra near it can react by sliding out of place.

Treatment: See your doctor or a physiatrist for either spondylolysis or spondylolisthesis. She'll order an X-ray or bone scan. Then she can see if you have a fractured or a slipped vertebra, and rate the degree of slippage. She might prescribe rest, or physical therapy, or possibly a brace. You will need to modify your athletic activities as you heal; for example, you might have to stop playing sports that call for a lot of back extension, such as gymnastics. For sports such as basketball and football, you might be able to modify your movements to protect your spine. Healing typically takes four months. Self-help methods of therapy include the following:

- Using heat or ice (see the box "Ice or Heat?" above).
- Taking OTC pain-relief medications. If OTC medication doesn't alleviate pain, your doctor might prescribe prescription medications. (See Chapter 9 for information about OTC and prescription medications.)

- Practicing meditation (see Chapter 6).
- Using exercises that stretch and strengthen your low back and its surrounding muscles (see Chapter 4).

If you have spondylolisthesis with no neurologic symptoms—that is, you have only low-back pain—your doctor might recommend physical or occupational therapy, or movement therapies including yoga, Pilates, tai chi, the Feldenkrais Method, or the Alexander Technique to alleviate your pain (see Chapter 5 for information about each of these therapies). Severe cases of spondylolisthesis—exhibiting neurologic symptoms and quite unstable vertebra—require spinal fusion surgery. Decompression surgery might be part of this surgical intervention, too. For information about surgical options, see Chapter 9.

SCIATIC NERVE PAIN

Symptoms: With classic sciatica, pain radiates from the back, down the leg, and sometimes into the calf or foot. It can cause tingling, numbness, or weakness (*neurologic symptoms*) in the leg. See your doctor as soon as possible if you are experiencing neurologic symptoms, which can also include bowel or bladder incontinence. He'll want to rule out cauda equina syndrome or other conditions associated with red flag symptoms.

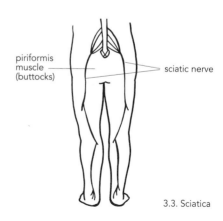

piriformis
muscle
(buttocks)

sciatic nerve

3.3. Sciatica

Explanation: Often you'll hear talk that makes sciatica sound like an actual disease. Instead, sciatica is a symptom and condition that can stem from various problems. The sciatic nerve runs from the lower back, traveling through both buttocks, down each thigh, with branches all the way down the legs into the feet. It wins the award for the largest nerve in the body. It's about as thick as one of your fingers.

Causes: The sciatic nerve can be irritated, impinged, or compressed for several different reasons. Simple causes include awkward sitting postures and muscle spasms including spasms of the piriformis muscle (see the Piriformis Syndrome section later in this chapter). Material from a disk herniation can affect the nerve roots. If the foramen (the hole the nerve goes through) is being narrowed, this can affect the nerve, too. This narrowing could be from osteoarthritis, degenerative disk disease, facet joint syndrome, spinal stenosis, or spondylolisthesis. Rarely, infections or tumors can be the root cause of sciatica.

Treatment: If you have sciatica, trying to find the root of the problem is essential. See your primary care physician or a physiatrist. He'll want to rule out any red flag symptoms and help you find the cause. Once you find the root cause—whether it is muscle spasms or spondylolisthesis—refer to related sections in this book for treatment options.

OTHER LOW-BACK PROBLEMS

Spinal Stenosis

Spinal stenosis is the technical term for the narrowing of the spinal canal. As the spinal canal gets skinnier, sometimes a nerve or nerve roots can become irritated or pinched. Spinal stenosis can occur for several reasons, including degenerative disk disease, the ligaments near the canal growing larger, and/or a genetic predisposition. Usually this condition affects people over the age of fifty. When you see an older person bending forward while walking, often they are doing this because it opens up the joints around the spinal canal, making it easier to walk. It is more comfortable for a person with spinal stenosis to sit as opposed to standing or walking.

Facet Joint Syndrome

The facet joints of each vertebral body connect the bone to the vertebrae above and below it and help move the spine in a controlled manner. A condition that typically affects people over the age of thirty-five, *facet joint syndrome* means that one or more facet joints are painful, usually worse with arching or twisting the body. This pain might mean there is fluid in the joints. Usually changes from osteoarthritis make the facet joints hurt in the same manner that an arthritic hip hurts.

Piriformis Syndrome

The piriformis muscle, which runs from the sacrum in the buttocks and attaches at the hip near the top of each femur bone, helps rotate the hip. The term *piriformis syndrome* stems from cadaver studies. Usually part of the sciatic nerve is located next to this muscle, but in a very small percentage of

THE LIST GOES ON AND ON

Numerous back books and articles list a plethora of diseases and conditions that can cause low-back pain. This can seem strange after you understand how hard it is pinpoint lumbar spine pain. Beyond the problems discussed in this chapter, it is helpful to recognize a few other conditions that can make your back ache. A chronic condition called **fibromyalgia,** which can cause fatigue, sleep problems, general body stiffness, and anxiety, also might cause pain and tenderness in your back. If you fall on your tailbone, or coccyx, located at the very bottom of the backbone, you can break your tailbone. A broken tailbone is called **coccydynia**. **Scoliosis**, a condition that means the spine curves to the side, usually does not cause pain. **Lordosis**— where the lumbar spine curve is exaggerated—can strain the back. Women can suffer from **gynecological problems** that cause back pain. Women with low-back pain should think about having a gynecological exam. Several non-musculoskeletal problems, such as kidney stones, might also be the cause of back pain. In other words, see your primary care physician for a physical exam. There are many conditions and diseases to consider when a patient complains of low-back pain.

cadavers, the muscle is split and the sciatic nerve passes through this division. If the piriformis muscle is too tight, it can compress the sciatic nerve and cause sciatic symptoms. Piriformis syndrome is a controversial topic, as some doctors don't believe it is an appropriate diagnosis. Other doctors say a person suffers from this syndrome when there is a tender piriformis muscle and radiating sciatic nerve pain. Runners, bikers, and athletes who do primarily forward movement with their legs without lateral movement tend to get piriformis syndrome. (If you swim the breaststroke, you will be including lateral movement, versus running, where you do mostly forward movement.) It's important to exercise in a balanced way.

Sacroiliac Joint Syndrome

The sacroiliac joint connects the low back to the pelvis, transferring weight from the lower back to the legs. This joint is involved every time we take a step. As with piriformis syndrome, *sacroiliac joint syndrome* is a heavily debated topic. The syndrome doesn't show up on X-rays, and some practitioners question whether it is the joint that is actually hurting. Some doctors believe sacroiliac joint syndrome means the joint is rotating backward or forward or slipping up or down a bit. The joint can be injured after a fall or a severe twisting motion. Diseases such as psoriatic arthritis and ankylosing spondylitis can affect the joint. Pregnant women or women who have given birth can also have sacroiliac joint problems because the ligaments and muscles around the joint loosen in preparation for childbirth.

Spinal Fracture

Stepping on a crack won't break your back (or your mother's back). It usually takes a significant trauma to break one or more vertebral bones. If you

THE TOOLBOX FOR LOW-BACK PAIN

Taking responsibility for your low-back pain means looking at the avenues to healing and deciding what might work for you. If you have a toolbox of ideas and supplies to deal with your pain, it probably looks different from your neighbor's toolbox. If a practitioner created a low-back toolbox for you, it would also be unique. Care providers all have their own beliefs and educational biases about what will alleviate or perhaps cure low-back problems. Still, the following "tools" for pain management might help you create a plan for your own back issue:

- Achieve the best possible level of fitness, including making lifestyle changes such as quitting smoking or drinking.
- Maintain that fitness level and those lifestyle changes.
- Explore whether the medicines you are taking right now are helping or harming you (for example, opiates can actually cause more pain).
- Accept the need to relieve stress.
- Accept the need to resolve conflict problems in relationships.
- Develop a multidisciplinary approach to healing—more than one therapy can be used for healing purposes.
- Be willing to explore the psychological aspects of chronic pain.
- Educate yourself about your condition and the therapies and bodyworks that might help.

fall from a high ladder and land on your spinal column, you might break one or more vertebral bones. A severe car crash can impact your spinal column, breaking vertebral bones. You might suffer a broken vertebral bone—called a *spinal fracture*—if you have a frail spine due to another condition, such as osteoporosis or cancer. Elderly people are much more likely to fracture the vertebrae in their backbones. If you fracture a vertebral bone, you will know right away that something is very wrong with your back. Seek medical attention immediately. Symptoms of spinal fractures include pain that lasts for more than two weeks, intense pain that interrupts your sleep, and pain that increases when you are actively moving.

LIVING WITH BACK PAIN

The back problems described in this chapter are classified as acute, subacute, or chronic back problems based on how long the pain persists. While labels can help us frame problems in our mind, you might wonder what you call the low-back strain that keeps reoccurring. The first time this back problem put you out of commission for a few days was two summers ago. Now you experience this pain a couple of times a year. Some practitioners would label this an acute flare-up of pain. It doesn't really matter what you call it. If you have re-occurring low-back problems, though, learning how to ease pain and finding tools to prevent this specific injury is a good idea. If you have daily lumbar spine pain, finding relief is foremost in your mind.

Maybe you've gone from one doctor to the next trying to find a solution, with little luck. Instead of thinking of professionals as the people with the solution for your back pain, place yourself in charge of your back problem.

Whether you experience acute bouts of pain that happen occasionally or chronic daily pain, learn to self-manage your condition. "The patient should, if at all possible, maintain a locus of control, educating themselves about their condition, using self-directed care measures, and occasionally checking in with the [medical] system," says Dr. Stan Herring, spine specialist at the University of Washington in Seattle.

Back pain is ultimately about management. Because each person is unique, solutions to back pain can take countless forms. Remember to think of all the various forms of treatments as spokes on a wheel. You are standing on the center hub, deciding which therapies might work for your ailment. In the following chapters, we'll discuss a plethora of options for back pain relief and healing. It's up to you to decide which one might work for your lifestyle. While yoga might be extremely advantageous for one person, physical therapy might be the best option for you. The great news: you can benefit from more than one of the numerous therapies that we'll explore in these pages. It's like going to your favorite store. On any given shopping trip, you'll find several items you want to try on for size, and possibly buy.

4 STRETCH YOUR BODY

OUR BODIES WERE MADE TO MOVE. We are not sedentary creatures. Long ago, we did not spend all our time sitting by the fire. When we are injury free, an all-day kayaking trip makes us feel more alive. Perhaps playing tennis with your kids is your favorite Saturday afternoon activity. Even though mowing the grass is a chore, there is some pleasure in pushing the mower across the blades of green grass.

You might stop your weekly kayak trip, though, if you have a low-back injury. The grass in your yard might grow long, and your children might miss playing tennis with you. While resting can be vital for recovery, usually that means *relative* rest. After an acute injury incident, temporarily avoiding activities that cause your back to hurt is vital, but you still can participate in your daily life. Moving your body is a key part of healing. It restores blood flow to the tissues, prevents the muscles, ligaments, and tendons from becoming deconditioned, and helps elevate your mood.

With chronic low-back pain, sometimes the back—or even the whole body—has gotten out of shape. Becoming more active can promote healing and help alleviate pain. Perhaps the yearly Thanksgiving tackle-football game is currently out of the question, but adding stretches to your after-dinner routine is a good idea.

In this chapter, you'll find numerous exercises designed to prevent low-back injuries. We've also included gentle stretches for easing lumbar spine pain, whether that hurt is acute or chronic. But first, we'll take a look at the way you move during your daily life, from how you pick up your kayak or forty-pound backpack to how you sit at your desk while working on your computer.

Important note: If you've never performed the stretches described in the following sections, please work with a trained professional first. An occupational therapist, physical therapist, or a professional trained in exercise physiology can show you the correct way to position your body and complete each exercise. Then you can perform these stretches on your own, with no danger of hurting yourself. See Chapter 5, "Finding a Movement Professional," for information about locating experts in these respective fields.

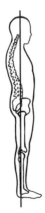

STAND UP STRAIGHT!

Can you hear your mom's voice in your head, reminding you not to slouch? She had your best interests in mind. Poor posture is one of the top contenders for causes of musculoskeletal disorders. Good posture means your body parts are in balance. The gentle S-curve of the spine is not overly exaggerated. The muscles are strong and flexible, especially the abdomen, hip, and leg muscles. Imagine a side view of a person with good posture—you would be able to draw a line through the ear, shoulder, hip, knee, and ankle.

You can check your posture at home. Evaluate your standing posture with the following tests from the American Physical Therapy Association:

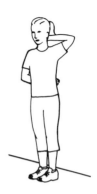

To check for normal curves of the spine:
- Stand with your back to a wall, heels about three inches from the wall.
- Place one hand behind your neck, with the back of the hand against the wall, and the other hand behind your low back with the palm against the wall.

If there is excessive space between your back and the wall, such that you can easily move your hands forward and back more than one inch, some adjustment in your posture may be necessary to restore the normal curves of your spine.

To check your posture from a front view, stand directly in front of a full-length mirror and answer the following questions:
- Is my head held straight (good posture) or does my head tilt to one side or another (bad posture)?
- Are my shoulders level (good posture) or is one shoulder lower than the other (bad posture)?
- Are the spaces between my sides and arms equal (good posture) or are the spaces unequal (bad posture)?
- Are my hips level (good posture) or is one hip higher than the other (bad posture)?

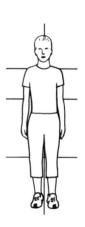

- Do my kneecaps face straight ahead (good posture) or do either of my knees turn in or out (bad posture)?
- Are my ankles straight (good posture) or do my ankles roll in so that the weight is on the inside of my feet (bad posture)?

If you find your posture lacking, this could be contributing to your low-back pain. Your primary care doctor can also evaluate your posture, or she might send you to a physical therapist for further review. Through physical therapy treatment, postural issues are corrected by building muscle strength and flexibility and learning the best way to stand, sit, and walk. You can also learn better postural traits through movement therapies including the Feldenkrais Method, the Alexander Technique, Pilates, tai chi, and yoga (see Chapter 5 for information about each of these movement therapies).

LIFTING 101

Often you've completed a task so many times that you no longer think about how you move your body. You hoist your eighty-pound canoe and carry it to the water. You lift your twenty-five-pound toddler into the air. Everyday tasks, right? So why does your back hurt?

So many motions can add stress to the lumbar spine, from lifting boxes and carrying children to toting groceries and planting flower bulbs. The fact is, thanks to gravity, the simple act of standing exerts force on your lumbar spine. For a man who is five foot nine and roughly one-hundred seventy-five pounds, gravity puts eighty pounds of compressive force on his lower back. Now he picks up a twenty-pound box and holds it ten inches from his body. This creates an additional one-hundred seventy pounds of pressure on his lower back. Ouch. How can you avoid straining your back while simply living your life?

It is all about *how* you perform everyday duties. Pick up your kayak correctly and you protect your back. Do the same task incorrectly and you strain your back. By performing the basic squat lift correctly, as illustrated below, you can lift moderate loads without stressing your lower back. If you are unfamiliar with performing the lifts described below, see Chapter 5, "Finding a Movement Professional," to find a professional to help you get it right.

The Squat Lift

1. Stand close to and face the object you are about to lift.
2. Bend your knees, not your back, and squat down.
3. Keep your back straight and firmly grasp the object.
4. Tighten your stomach muscles, pick up the object, and hold it close to the center of your body.
5. Stand up slowly, letting your leg muscles do the carrying work.
6. Never twist while you lift the object; turn with your legs if you need to pivot.

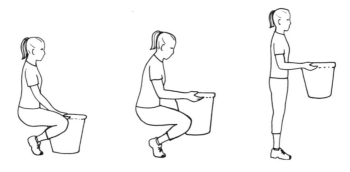

The Partial Golf Pick-Up

Have you ever watched a golfer pick up a golf ball? Usually she lifts one leg off the ground while picking up the ball. Use the partial golf pick-up to retrieve your groceries from the car trunk or to grab that tennis ball that landed in the bushes. Even though these objects aren't always heavy, your back will thank you for moving wisely as you reach for them.

1. When lifting from a car trunk, place one leg on the bumper. Keep your back straight and slide the object to the edge of the car trunk.
2. Before lifting the object, place both feet on the ground.
3. Place one hand on the car (or washing machine, etc.).
4. Reach in with the other arm, keeping the back straight, and pivot from the hips while extending the opposite leg backwards.
5. Grasp the object firmly, and slowly lift while straightening at the hips, pushing with the other arm and bringing the leg back down.
6. Position the object close to the center of the body.

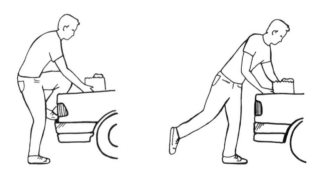

The Full Golf Pick-Up

If you are lifting an object that weighs a pound or less, you can use a full golf pick-up lift. If you currently have back pain, have had back surgery, or you are pregnant, avoid this lift.

1. Keeping the back straight, pivot at the hips while extending one leg straight behind you as you reach down to pick up the object.
2. As you pivot back up with the object, swing the straight leg back down.

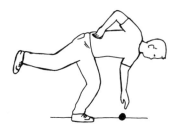

WORKSTATION 101

Many of us spend our workday at a computer station. Perhaps you read the news online now. Many of us spend plenty of our free time on the Internet, emailing and instant messaging friends, and looking for new hiking locales and cheap flights for our next adventure. Sitting in a chair—even if a screen is not in front of you—is more stressful on your lower back than standing upright or lying down. If your lower back is unsupported while sitting, often your body responds by slouching. This puts even more pressure on your lumbar spine and its disks. Low-back pain can be a direct result of poor sitting posture.

Have you ever heard the term *neutral posture*? This simply means you are in the most natural, relaxed position for your body. Think about how your body feels as you float in a lake: this is your neutral posture. When you are in this position, your body parts are well balanced, down to the right amount of space between your spinal column's vertebral bones. Using a well-designed chair can promote your best posture; ask your occupational or physical therapist for chair recommendations. Neutral posture chairs made by Neutral Posture, Inc., have won ergonomic awards (see "Resources" at the back of this book).

No matter what type of office chair you choose, using the following sitting and computer-work suggestions can prevent and ease strain on your low back.

Sitting in a Chair

- Your hips should be slightly higher than your knees, or equal height to your knees. Pick the one that feels best to you.
- Your feet should be flat on the floor.
- If you are working at a computer, your chair back should be slightly reclined, about 10 to 20 degrees, so you feel the space between your torso and your hips opening up a little bit.
- The chair back's curve should offer support at your lumbar or low spine. If not, add a rolled-up towel or a lumbar support pillow to support your natural back curve.

Working at a Computer

- Your elbows should be close to your body; this might mean not using the chair's armrests.

- Your hands should be level with your elbows, or a little below your elbows.
- Your wrists should be straight, with the forearms and hands in a straight line.
- You shouldn't have to reach too far for any item while working. Your mouse should be the same height as your keyboard and immediately next to your keyboard, within easy reach.

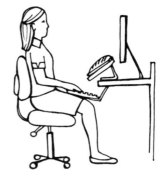

- Your shoulders should be relaxed. Sometimes using armrests can tighten up your shoulders.
- The computer screen should be eighteen to twenty-eight inches away, at eye-level or a little below eye-level.

If you find that sitting at a computer desk for hours strains your back, regardless of sitting in an ergonomically correct posture, try standing for part of your workday. You can stand while making phone calls—if you don't need to look at your monitor or type at the same time. You can also create a standing workstation. The ideal height for your keyboard and monitor depends on your height. Your computer screen should be at or just below eye-level. While you type, you should be able to maintain a comfortable body position with your shoulders relaxed at your side. Make sure your elbows are bent between 70 to 90 degrees and keep your wrists straight.

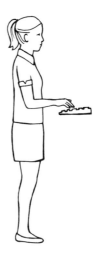

Another alternative to sitting in a chair is to use a fitness ball for short bursts of time. Sitting on a fitness ball does help build your core muscle tone and encourages you to vary your posture. However, sitting on a fitness ball is tiring, and it doesn't mean you will use your best posture. If you are not having an acute bout of back pain, you can experiment with using a fitness ball. Perhaps super-fit competitive-level athletes can perch on fitness balls all day long, but most of us should work on a fitness ball for small "breaks" during office hours, adding up to roughly an hour or two.

Work Break Stretches

Good posture is also about varying movement. Seattle-area occupational therapist Carolyn Salazar, MS, tells her patients, "Your next posture is your best posture." Changing your position promotes blood flow and gets your muscles moving.

While this means making slight variations while you are standing or sitting, or getting up from sitting and taking a short walk once an hour, it's also vital to stretch throughout the workday. A study published in 2004 by the *European Journal of Applied Physiology and Occupational Physiology* found that "micropauses" can provide an immediate sense of relief and postpone the threshold for fatigue. A *micropause* is a short break of three to five seconds. Look away from the computer toward a spot in the distance and lift your hands off the keyboard to ease tension. Do this about every ten minutes. Micropauses can also ease eyestrain and prevent computer-related injury. If stopping every ten minutes seems unlikely, try taking a three- to five-minute stretch break once an hour.

Often, moving your body in exactly the opposite way is helpul. If you are sitting in front of a computer, stand and do a backward bend. The lumbar rotation exercise can ease low-back stiffness.

Backward Bend

1. Stand with your feet hip-distance apart.
2. Place your hands on your hips.
3. Arch backward to make the hollow of your back deeper.
4. Hold for three to five seconds.

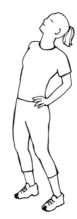

Lumbar Rotation

1. While sitting, cross your arms and place each hand on its opposite shoulder.
2. Gently rotate your trunk from side to side in a small, pain-free range of motion.

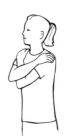

You can set a timer on your watch to remind yourself to take stretch breaks, or download various computer programs that will remind you to take periodic breaks. A popular program called "Stretch Break" has a computer-generated person perform stretches so you can simply follow along (see "Resources" at the back of the book).

At the end of a long workday, or before going to sleep, stretch out your lower back again:

Knee-to-Chest Stretch

1. Lie on your back on the floor. Place your right hand behind your right knee.
2. Pull this knee in toward your chest until you feel a comfortable stretch in your lower back and buttocks. Keep your back relaxed.
3. Hold for five seconds. Repeat with your left knee.

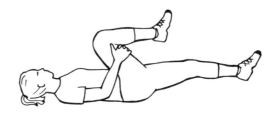

Lower Trunk Rotation Stretch

1. Lie on the floor with your back flat.
2. With your feet together, rotate your knees to the right side.
3. Hold for three to five seconds. Repeat, this time rotating your knees to the left side.

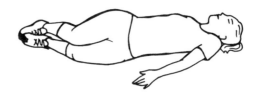

MOVE YOUR BODY EVERY DAY

Don't let back pain stop you from being active—exercise is part of the cure. Of course, if you suffer from low-back pain, you should check with your health-care provider before embarking on a new exercise regimen. Exercising on a regular basis is probably the most important activity you can do. Regular aerobic activity helps promote good posture and better sleep; increases the strength, endurance, and flexibility of muscles and other connective tissues; elevates your mood; decreases depression and anxiety; and helps manage stress.

It's ideal to move your body every day. Although you'll want to start off slowly and follow your doctor's guidelines, healthy adults under the age of sixty-five need thirty minutes of moderately intense physical exercise at least five times a week to stay in good health, according to recommendations released by the American College of Sports Medicine and the American Heart Association in 2007. How should you feel if you are working out at a moderate rate? You'll break a sweat and raise your heart rate, but you can still talk to your jogging partner.

If you sit at work all day, take walk breaks during office hours to counteract the effects of sitting. Before or after work, go for a swim, a bike ride, or a long walk. Even if you have a physical job, usually you are not engaged aerobically during your workday. To get that blood pumping, go for a run or schedule a squash game in the evening. If your job involves standing for the better part of eight hours, a bike ride or a swim will stretch and exercise your body in different ways. Even if you go kayaking or hiking every weekend, you need to fit in aerobic activities during the week.

Vary your aerobic activities for the best results. Swim one day, bicycle on another, run or speed walk on another day. This cross-training will

STRENGTH & FLEXIBILITY TRAINING

Maybe you have never been a gym rat. Perhaps you prefer exercising in the great outdoors or in the comfort of your home. If you don't visit a fitness club, there's a good chance you aren't lifting weights or doing resistance training. This type of work builds muscle mass and increases bone density. Strength training makes a body strong, aiding in the prevention of injury and helping the body deal more effectively with injury when it occurs. Ideally, a person should lift weights or work on resistance training for thirty minutes, two to three nonconsecutive days a week. A physical therapist, certified personal trainer, or a professional trained in exercise physiology can help you create a strength-training regimen.

develop a variety of muscles groups and help muscles develop in a more complete way.

Feel too tired to exercise? Don't believe it. A University of Georgia study published in 2008 examined whether exercise could be used to treat fatigue. The fatigued participants engaged in either low- or high-intensity workouts three times a week for six weeks. At the end of the six weeks, they found that regular exercise had increased their energy levels by 20 percent. The study also found that the exercisers who participated in a low-intensity workout felt a 65 percent drop in tiredness, while the group doing more intense exercise felt only a 49 percent drop in fatigues. So taking an easy stroll after a long day might be even better than going for an intense, long run.

STRETCHES TO STRENGTHEN YOUR LOWER BACK

Does stretching before a workout prevent injury? Results from studies on this question are inconclusive. However, a study published in 2005 in Norway showed that a pre-workout warm-up that included *dynamic* exercises did help prevent injuries.

What's the difference between static and dynamic stretches and exercises? Simple stretching is usually a static movement: you slowly move your body until you experience a mild pulling sensation and then you hold the stretch for twenty to thirty seconds. Static stretches are probably best at the end of a workout (unless you are doing an exercise that requires a lot of flexibility, such as gymnastics or ballet).

Dynamic movement, on the other hand, means stretching the body while moving. In a dynamic warm-up, you move through a series of the motions you will use during your workout. This helps loosen muscles and tendons and increases the range of motion in various joints. Dynamic movement stretches can be helpful because they help warm up your muscles.

An aerobic warm-up, such as running for about five to ten minutes and then resting for five minutes before you work out, will literally warm you up, increasing blood circulation and body heat.

An aerobic warm-up can also mean performing dynamic exercises. American College of Sports Medicine (ACSM) personal trainer Sebastien Alary recommends completing a few of the following exercises before your workouts. All of these active, dynamic stretches will help strengthen and stretch out your lower back and the surrounding muscles. Although each stretch is described for one side of the body, do each stretch bilaterally. For example, after your right leg is in the bent knee position, do the stretch with your left knee bent. (If you have never practiced stretches similar to those described below, see Chapter 5, "Finding a Movement Professional," for information about finding a professional practitioner who can instruct you in how to perform these movement therapies.)

Exercise Ball QL Muscles Stretch

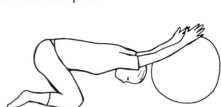

1. Lie on the floor on your right side. Lean your upper body on an exercise ball, with your right elbow on the ball and bent.
2. Stretch out your right leg so it is lying straight along the floor.
3. Place your left foot—with the knee bent—flat on the floor in front of your right leg. Focus on pulling your upper body away from your right leg. This stretches your right *quadratus lumborum* muscle, which is one link between the pelvis and the spine.

Exercise Ball Lats Stretch

1. Kneel in front of an exercise ball with your knees about shoulder-width apart.
2. Extend both arms in front of you and place your hands— palms facing toward each other—on either side of an exercise ball.
3. Lower your head and focus on stretching your upper body and low back. You will feel a stretch in your back's *latissimus dorsi* muscles, which are one link between the spine and the pelvis.

Plank Walk

1. Stand with your feet shoulder distance apart. Bend from your waist and place your hands on the ground in front of you so your body makes about a 45-degree angle.
2. Walk your feet toward your hands. Do not force a stretch, just walk toward your hands and feel a light to moderate stretch in your hamstring muscles.
3. Move your hands farther out again, so your body makes roughly a 45-degree angle, and walk your feet toward your hands again. Do this stretch a handful of times.

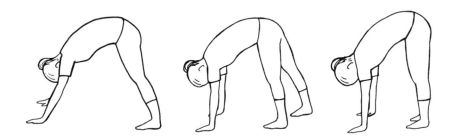

Exercise Ball Front and Back Balance Stretches

1. Lie face down on an exercise ball, with your elbows and hands on the floor in front of you and your toes on the floor behind you.
2. Roll back and forth, moving the ball along the upper front of your body.
3. Next, lie with your back on the ball. Place your feet flat on the floor and extend your arms out to either side. Let your head fall back and relax.

4. Roll back and forth, moving the ball along your spine. Both of these stretches also feel good, giving your back a gentle massage.

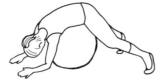 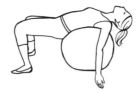

Medicine Ball Movements

1. Stand with your feet apart, wider than the hips, with feet facing forward. Bend your knees.
2. Extend your arms in front of you while holding a medicine ball. (Make sure the medicine ball doesn't weigh too much, as you need to move this weighted ball.)
3. Now move the ball in a number of ways: up and down, back and forth, and in circles. You can even move your hips as you move the ball, or point a toe to the side and bend one knee at a time. Find a movement you really like and practice this movement.

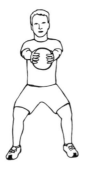 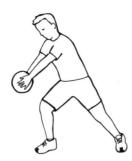

STRETCHES FOR PREVENTING LOW-BACK PAIN

After a workout, your muscles are warmed up and capable of greater movement with less effort. By performing static stretches after your workout, you can more effectively lengthen a group of muscles, making muscles and connective tissues more flexible and less injury-prone. Muscles, tendons, ligaments, and joints that have a greater range of motion are not as likely to strain or tear when they are warmed up.

"Any exercise shortens or tightens muscles. What's really important is to do as much stretching as you are exercising," says Laura Yon-Brook, MA, LMP, RYT, a sports-medicine professional and yoga teacher who has worked with professional athletes. Stretching and lengthening muscles helps keep them flexible and strong. If you don't stretch immediately after exercising, spend time stretching in the evening after your muscles are warm from the day's activities.

Physical therapist Wolfgang Brolley, founder of Stretch Physical Therapy in Seattle, recommends the following stretches for preventing low-back pain. Although each stretch is described for one side of the body, do each stretch bilaterally. For example, after your right leg is in the bent knee position, do the stretch with your left knee bent. (If you have never practiced stretches similar to those described below, see Chapter 5, "Finding a Movement Professional," for information about finding a professional practitioner who can instruct you in how to perform these movement therapies.)

In the exercises that follow, *neutral spine* means your spine is essentially in a position that feels natural and comfortable to you. A physical therapist or exercise specialist can help you find this position. Alternatively, while standing, move your backbone and tilt your pelvis in various positions, seeing what feels best.

Hip Flexor Stretch

1. Put one foot up on a counter or other solid edge that is about the height of your hips.
2. Stand with a neutral spine and with your other foot slightly behind you.
3. Tilt your pelvis and then push your hips toward the counter while holding neutral spine.

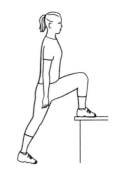

Hip Adductor Stretch

1. Sit with your back against a wall, your knees bent at a right angle, and the arches of your feet together.
2. Maintain a neutral spine while using your hands to push gently down on your knees.
3. Hold for five to ten breaths.

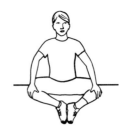

Hamstring Stretch

1. Lying on your back, clasp both hands behind one bent leg and straighten the other leg onto the floor.
2. Pull gently on your bent leg while slowly straightening the knee. You will feel a gentle stretch. (It's not necessary to straighten the knee and leg fully.)

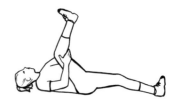

Quadriceps Stretch 1

1. Lie on your stomach with your belly button centered on a pillow.
2. Bend one knee, grasp the ankle with your hand (or use a belt), and pull your heel toward your buttocks.

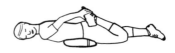

Quadriceps Stretch 2

1. Hook the top of your foot behind you on a desk.
2. Keeping neutral spine, bend your opposite knee.
3. For a higher level of stretch, keep the knee of the stretched leg behind your hip.

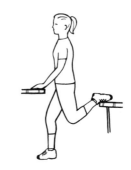

Iliotibial Band/Piriformis Stretch 1

1. While lying on your back, bend your right leg. Put your right hand behind your right knee and hold your right ankle with your left hand.
2. While maintaining a neutral spine, push your knee toward your opposite shoulder while pulling your ankle toward you.

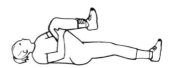

Iliotibial Band/Piriformis Stretch 2

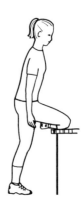

1. Stand on one leg, with your right leg bent at the knee at a 90-degree angle (your knee will be directly in front of your hip); rest your bent leg on a hip-height surface.

2. You will feel a stretch in your right piriformis muscle. If your knee is lying flat on the table and you want to feel a deeper stretch, lean forward from your hips while maintaining a neutral spine.

YOGA POSES TO STRETCH AND STRENGTHEN YOUR LOWER BACK

Yoga poses can stretch and strengthen your low back. If you have lumbar spine pain, get your doctor's approval before starting a yoga practice. Yoga is not meant to replace medical care, but is instead an adjunct therapy. If you are new to yoga, it's best to learn with a certified instructor, either in a one-on-one setting or in a beginner's class, perhaps one designed for people with low-back issues.

For the following poses, it is helpful but not necessary to place a pillow or block between your feet or knees and squeeze it; this helps you to contract your adductor and deep inner core muscles. You will be more comfortable on a yoga mat or at least on a rug. (If you never have practiced yoga poses similar to those described below, see Chapter 5, "Finding a Movement Professional," for information about finding a yoga instructor who can teach you how to perform these movement therapies correctly.)

Cat–Cow Flow

1. Start on your hands and knees in what is called the *table pose*. Your palms should be flat on the mat directly under your shoulders, your knees below your hips, and your feet stretched out. Your spine should be in a neutral position, with your back long—essentially in a position that feels natural to you.

2. Slowly inhale, lowering your mid-spine and belly while lifting your tailbone, chest, and heart upward. Look forward slightly.

3. Slowly exhale, rounding your back slowly upward (like a cat). Push your belly button toward the sky and tuck your chin in toward your chest.

4. Flow through this movement five to ten times, breathing deeply in and out. This flow gently wakes up and massages the spine.

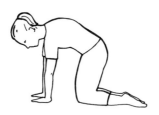 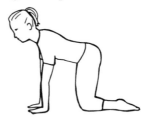

Table into Child Flow

1. Start on your hands and knees in the table pose, with your palms flat on the mat directly under your shoulders, your knees below your hips, and your feet stretched out. Your spine should be in a neutral position, with your back long—essentially in a position that feels natural to you.

A HOME MAINTENANCE ROUTINE

State Patrol Lieutenant Jeff Huettl, from rural Minnesota, isn't sure how he hurt his back, but he believes the injury was linked to poor posture and overexertion from activities such as cutting, splitting, moving, and stacking firewood as quickly as possible. He experienced his first symptoms while crouching and playing with his dog. Huettl has two bulging disks in the L4 and L5 vertebral sections, and a torn L5 disk. His rehabilitation doctor thinks Huettl underwent severe muscle spasms from overusing muscles that weren't sufficiently strong; in the doctor's mind, damage wasn't the real problem.

Huettl's initial treatment included bed rest, medication, cortisone injections, and physical therapy. His physical therapy team created a home maintenance program de-signed to prevent future flare-ups of pain. This exercise regimen included ten prevention stretches and four exercises; some of them were supposed to be performed twice a day, others a few times a week. Huettl admits, though, that he completes his stretches just once a day and his exercises not quite as often as he should.

Since his initial recovery, Huettl has had smaller reoccurrences of pain. These happened when he hadn't been doing his stretching and exercising on a regular basis, and when he overexerted himself, spending a full day chopping firewood, for example. Huettl has found that his home maintenance routine really keeps the hurt at bay, as does doing his exercises and stretches before and after he completes any physical work.

2. Slowly exhale, lowering your tailbone to your heels, extending your arms, and tucking your head so your eyes face downward. You will feel a gentle stretch in your shoulders. This is called *child's pose*.
3. Slowly inhale, lifting your tailbone from your heels and shifting forward until you are back in the table position.
4. Flow through this movement five to ten times while breathing deeply in and out.

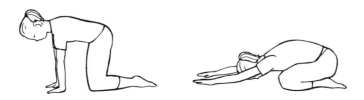

Sphinx

1. Lie on the mat with your elbows on the floor and your hands in line with your ears. Rest one cheek on the floor.
2. Inhale slowly, pressing your pelvis and feet into the mat, originating the movement from your low back. Keeping your hands, forearms, and elbows on the floor, peel your chest off the floor and pull forward slightly with your hands, lifting your gaze to center and slightly forward.
3. Exhale slowly, reversing the movement, ending up with your opposite cheek resting on the mat.
4. Repeat this movement five to ten times, so each cheek has rested on the floor the same number of times.

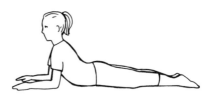

Low Cobra

1. Lie on your mat with your palms facing down under your shoulders, elbows tucked in and off the floor. Rest one cheek on the floor.
2. Inhale slowly, pressing your pelvis and feet into the floor, originating the movement from your low back. Peel your chest off the floor while keeping your hands on the ground below your shoulders and your elbows tucked in, lifting your gaze to center and slightly forward. Squeeze your thighs together as you lift.
3. Exhale slowly, reversing the movement, ending up with your opposite cheek resting on the mat.
4. Repeat the movement five to ten times, so each check has rested on the floor the same number of times.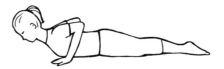

Standing Hip Circles

1. Stand with your feet hip-distance apart. Bend your knees and place your hands on your hips.
2. Inhale slowly, pulling your belly in and tightening the core abdominal muscles.
3. Exhale slowly, feeling your body relaxing and picturing your shoulders dropping away from your ears.
4. Rotate your hips in first a clockwise and then a counter-clockwise direction, taking five seconds to complete each circle.
5. Do hip circles ten times, with five hip circles in each direction.

5 FINDING A MOVEMENT PROFESSIONAL

SOMETIMES YOU CAN MANAGE LOW-BACK PAIN without the help of professionals. Perhaps your back is out-of-whack after a weekend of rock climbing. You take ibuprofen, ice your lumbar spine every four hours, spend extra time stretching, and watch how you move. After a few days of self-care, your pain dissipates.

Other bouts of back pain can leave you wondering who to call for help. Perhaps you took a bad tumble while snowboarding and then found yourself curled up in the fetal position for the better part of three days. Or, as the parent of two children under the age of three, you've found that your lumbar spine pain has become progressively worse. Now stabs of radiating pain and a crying baby interrupt your sleep.

What low-back health-care practitioner can ease you hurt and start you on the road to healing? In this chapter, we'll talk about professionals who help people with acute, subacute, or chronic low-back pain start moving on the road to recovery.

THE ROLE OF A PHYSIATRIST

When your back goes out, often the first person you call is your primary care doctor. Next time, you might want to consider booking an appointment with a physiatrist as well. A *physiatrist (fi-zē-á-trist)*, also called a *rehabilitation physician,* is a nerve, muscle, and bone expert trained in physical medicine and rehabilitation. As specialists in treating illnesses and injuries that affect how people move their bodies, physiatrists are especially well qualified to deal with back injuries.

Find a physiatrist who specializes in back pain or musculoskeletal problems. He will look at the functional side of your low-back pain. In addition to talking about your symptoms, he'll discuss what you were doing when you hurt your back, how the pain is affecting your daily life, and what activities you can't do that you want or need to do. (You should also discuss these issues with your primary care doctor.)

The physiatrist might prescribe several types of treatments, such as medication, injections, chiropractic or osteopathic treatments, massage therapy, or physical therapy. He will most likely have you begin a self-activated exercise program, such as walking every day. Physiatrists believe in educating patients about their conditions and helping patients understand that movement is an important tool for easing low-back pain.

Before making an appointment with a physiatrist, check with your health insurance. Your insurance company might require that you get a referral from your primary care physician.

THE ROLE OF PHYSICAL THERAPY

If you are experiencing acute, subacute, or chronic back pain, you may need to relearn how to perform daily chores and work- or recreation-related activities in ways that don't harm your low back. Relearning some movements can help diminish your hurt. A physical therapist can show you how to complete chores such as doing the laundry, carrying your toddler on a hike, portaging a canoe between lakes, or moving heavy equipment around your work place in ways that protect your lumbar spine. Often your primary care provider or physiatrist will prescribe appointments with a physical therapist. Usually a doctor's referral ensures that your health insurance will pay for this therapy, but some states do allow patients to see a physical therapist without a doctor's prescription. Like physiatrists, physical therapists have studied physical rehabilitation and work with patients who have illnesses or injuries that limit their ability to move their bodies and perform both daily and leisure activities.

Physical therapists (PTs) approach a low-back problem from a functional point-of-view. According to the American Physical Therapy Association (see "Resources," at the back of this book), a PT will develop a treatment plan designed to improve your ability to move, reduce pain, restore function, and prevent disability. A PT will help you build up the strength, endurance, power, and coordination of the muscles and other connective tissues that support your lumbar spine.

Physical therapists focus on rehabilitating your low back and body. Sometimes this includes focusing on movements you employ in your daily, personal life—getting dressed, vacuuming the house, or picking up your toddler. Sometimes your work duties contribute to your pain: the way you sit at your desk, type on your keyboard, or complete repetitive tasks. Often a physical therapist will address all of these concerns, but you may need to see an occupational therapist as well. Sometimes occupational therapists work in tandem with physical therapists at larger clinics. An occupational

MULTIDISCIPLINARY CARE

Whether you suffer from acute, subacute, or chronic low-back pain, sometimes you need more than one type of practitioner to find relief. Perhaps you have a herniated disk from a snowboarding fall. When the pain medications failed to relieve your pain, you went to see an anesthesiologist for an epidural steroid injection. Once you started feeling better, a physical therapist created an exercise program that helped you achieve full range of motion in your low back. After you were able to exercise every day, you joined a weekly yoga class, adding another tool to your pain-prevention toolbox.

Technically speaking, you are receiving multidisciplinary care for your herniated disk.

The term *multidisciplinary care* takes on new meaning if you have been suffering from chronic pain for years. Often this daily hurt has touched every aspect of your life. Chronic-pain patients can seek care at a rehabilitation center, which means a place where all the multidisciplinary care happens under the umbrella of one practice. Taking a team approach to chronic low-back pain, physiatrists or pain-management physicians, physical therapists, occupational therapists, vocational counselors, psychologists, and bodyworks practitioners work together to help each individual patient.

When you participate in a multidisciplinary pain rehabilitation program, you work side-by-side daily for weeks with other people who are suffering from chronic pain. "Sharing the pain rehabilitation experience with people in similar situations can create therapeutic momentum," says Dr. J. David Sinclair, pain management specialist in Seattle, Washington. Group therapy provided for other chronic conditions has been shown to be beneficial; similarly, working with chronically impaired pain patients in pain management can create what is sometimes called "the magic of the group."

Sometimes insurance providers will not pay for care at a rehabilitation center. Still, you can piece together a rehabilitation team, seeking care from various providers yourself. By obtaining referrals from your primary care doctor, you might be able to gain insurance coverage for your piecemeal multidisciplinary care team.

therapist is a professional who teaches a patient how to apply safe body mechanics to everyday life from bathing, dressing, hygiene, and feeding, to high-level activities such as grocery shopping and driving. (Occupational therapists are often part of a hospital staff, teaching skills such as eating to patients such as stroke victims. Occupational therapists also work with disease and limits of the upper extremities, including the shoulders, elbows, wrists, and hands.) Some occupational therapists specialize in workplace settings; seek out this person to help you set up your office if your physical therapist is unable to assist you. The goal of both physical and occupational therapy is to help a patient become as independent as possible, completing daily living skills unaided.

Choosing a Physical Therapist

Often, your doctor will recommend a specific physical therapist. Several organizations can also point you in the right direction. With the American Physical Therapy Association's consumer website (see "Resources," at the back of this book), you can locate physical therapists by geographical location or by their advanced specialty degree.

Some physical therapists are trained in the *McKenzie Method,* also known as *Mechanical Diagnosis and Therapy*. These physical therapists perform an initial patient assessment that looks at how pain and symptoms relate to your movements; the therapist then uses this information to create a treatment plan. Another goal of McKenzie Method–trained therapists is to teach you how to be in control of your own back issues, so you can take care of yourself. You can locate a McKenzie Method–trained physical therapist at the McKenzie Institute's website (see "Resources," at the back of this book).

If you are seeking a physical therapist for acute, subacute, or chronic pain, look for an experienced physical therapist. This doesn't mean you need to seek out someone with twenty-five-plus years of experience. Instead, if your physical therapist is a recent graduate, ask if he is working in a clinic with a mentor program where newer therapists receive guidance from more experienced therapists.

You'll be seeing your physical therapist a lot, sometimes twice a week or more. You will want to feel comfortable with this person. Larger physical therapy offices often have assistants; you'll spend time with the physical therapist and part of each session with the assistant. Make sure you are at ease with the assistants as well, and that you can see the physical therapist when you feel it is necessary.

The First Appointment

If you have never seen a physical therapist, you might wonder how this appointment is different from a doctor's appointment. Every patient is unique, so the physical therapist won't be deciding on a treatment plan simply by reading your MRI or asking about your doctor's diagnosis. The physical therapist will ask you questions about how your pain behaves, and how it changes with your positions, movements, emotions, and social situations. The appointment will be very physical. The physical therapist will watch you move, observing how you sit, walk, and stand, and even how you sleep (your preferred positions). Most importantly, the physical therapist will be actually touching your body, both while you are in motion and at rest, to see how your body's parts move together and to check for injury as well as strength.

The physical therapist will also ask you what activities your back pain has forced you to curtail. The answers to this question will vary widely. Maybe you want to roughhouse with your children without wincing with pain, to run five times a week again, or to rejoin your Wednesday-night basketball league. Or perhaps you need help in finding a better way to work at your computer or a more comfortable sleeping position. The goals you describe will guide your physical therapy sessions. Your physical therapist will create an exercise program to strengthen your back so that playing with your kids is fun again or you can adopt an exercise program that leads to running or playing three-on-three basketball. She can also guide you in arranging your computer station or sleeping position correctly.

Physical Therapy Modalities

Physical therapists might use one or more *passive therapies*, or *modalities*, to help treat your injured back. Generally, the patient *receives* this treatment (that is, she is not actively involved in the treatment). Some physical therapists use these passive treatments sparingly, preferring patients to be as actively involved in their recovery as possible. Nonetheless, these modalities can help ease pain and promote healing. Often physical therapists use these modalities to treat the discomfort associated with acute pain or the acute flare-ups suffered by chronic back pain patients.

- **Heat** or **cold packs** can help relieve your pain. (For information on using heat or cold therapy at home, see the box "Ice or Heat?" in Chapter 3.)
- **Electrical stimulation** uses electrical current to cause a single muscle or a group of muscles to contract by putting electrodes on the skin. The muscles are either gently or forcefully contracted. This modality is often used for flare-ups of pain, sometimes in conjunction with an ice pack.

Electrical stimulation can also help retrain muscles and nerves to work together to move.

- **Transcutaneous Electrical Nerve Stimulation,** or **TENS,** also uses a low level of electrical stimulation (which does not stimulate contraction of the muscles) to disrupt an unrelenting pain cycle by temporarily blocking a pain message. Often used for chronic pain, TENS is not a curative. Some therapists use TENS in tandem with exercise therapy, and recommend learning how to ease pain through a cognitive behavior modification therapy program.
- **Ultrasound** is a short, deep-heat therapy that uses high-frequency sound waves. This eases pain, increases circulation, and relaxes tissues and muscles for a short duration, but at a deeper level than a heat pack.
- If you have a hard time doing land-based therapy, due to weight or movement issues, you might participate in **water therapy**. You'll complete exercises during active water therapy. When you are in a pool, gravity no longer exerts a force on your lumbar spine. If you have severe low-back pain, this can make it easier for you to complete movements. As you begin to heal, you might transition from water to a land-based regimen.
- If you experience excessive pain while moving, a **corset** or **brace** is a temporary fix. The corset or brace restricts movement while you learn muscle control and postures to ease this pain. This modality might be used after surgery. If you use a corset or brace for too long, however, muscles and other connective tissues become deconditioned because you rely on the corset or brace to help move your body.
- **Manual medicine** and **massage therapy** relieve pain and stimulate a healing response. Your physical therapist might use these modalities

when you plateau, meaning you are not getting any better or worse, to help jump-start the therapeutic process. The physical therapist or massage therapist uses their hands to localize the force on deep tissues and joints of the back and body. (For more information on massage therapy, turn to Chapter 7.)

Exercises and Physical Therapy

The bulk of each physical therapy appointment is about movement. The physical therapist will create a stretching and exercise regimen to address your low back's specific problems. Although each regimen is unique, often a patient will work on:

- Postural and gait issues.
- Strengthening core muscles, a large rectangle of muscles from your knees all the way to your neck, including abdominal and pelvic floor muscles, as well as the *multifidi*, *erector spinae*, and *iliopsoas* muscles.
- General aerobic conditioning to build endurance, bring oxygen to the tissues, and elevate mood. Often a daily walking regimen is recommended.
- Strength and resistance training to build the overall strength of the body.
- Relearning daily chores, activities, and sports techniques, so you can perform them in a way that doesn't harm your low back.

Your physical therapist is trying to improve the perceivable deficits caused by your low-back issues. This will mean performing exercises during appointments and doing exercises on a daily basis. Your physical therapist will break the exercises into steps or stages, teaching you how to perform each movement correctly, including breathing techniques. The exercises shouldn't provoke

CHRONIC PAIN AND MOVEMENT

If you are suffering from chronic low-back pain, you might experience pain while doing safe, therapeutic exercises. This feels wrong, but the hurt isn't causing any new damage. You are experiencing pain because the body has changed in response to chronic pain. The pain has been rerouted to a chronic pain pathway, which means the hurt is not coordinated with an anatomical issue. The physical therapy exercise might hurt, and the pain you feel is real, but that doesn't mean you shouldn't complete the exercise; you are working to lessen or change those chronic pain pathways. Ask your physical therapist to explain how chronic pain reroutes pain circuits. Understanding chronic pain will make it easier to work through the hurt. As your pain pathways change, you'll hurt less, and you'll also be learning to move in a way that is less painful.

symptoms, but you can expect soreness, similar to the pain you would feel from completing any exercise regimen. (You might continue doing some daily exercises for the rest of your life.) You'll learn how to move with the least amount of pain possible during your daily life and while participating in your favorite leisure activities.

YOGA

Moving your body is often the best thing you can do for yourself after a back injury. While this can mean moving your body through its daily routines, it also means exercising. According to recent studies, yoga can be a very beneficial form of exercise when you are suffering from low-back pain.

Although yoga originated in India, where people have been practicing it for centuries, it has also become a familiar part of our exercise culture in America. You are likely to find a yoga program at your local health club, in a nearby hospital or health center, at your community center, or in a neighbor's basement studio just down the street.

Perhaps you think yoga is only for flexible people. "Saying 'I can't do yoga because I'm not flexible' is like saying 'I can't take guitar lessons because I don't know how to play guitar,'" says Valerie Crosby, a certified yoga teacher in Albuquerque, New Mexico.

Yoga is about intentional movement. "It's the practice of moving the body with the breath," explains Cathy Prescott, a senior teacher and mentor for Integrative Yoga Therapy, who lives in Niskayuna, New York. "I talk with my hands, but this is not yoga. If I stop, take a breath, lift my arms, and exhale, that is yoga. I have to concentrate, breathe, and pay attention to the movement I make."

In India and the United States, developing self-understanding has always been one of the main principles of yoga. This self-understanding and unity is gained through yoga *poses* (also called *postures*, or *asanas*), as well as through breathing (*pranayama).* Sometimes yoga includes meditation (*dhyana*). While practicing yoga, you will move into various postures and use various breathing techniques. Doing this will stretch and strengthen your body and relax your mind. Intentional movement and breathing makes you aware of your body and helps place you in the present moment.

Yoga does not replace medical care; it is, instead, an adjunct treatment. Before you begin a yoga practice, check with your primary care physician to see if she feels you are ready to participate in yoga.

The Proof Is in the Practice

A study published in 2005 by the Group Health Research Institute in Seattle showed yoga to be more effective for low-back pain than conventional exercise. Twenty-six weeks into the study, the patients who completed twelve weekly gentle yoga classes had better back-related function and less pain than the participants who attended twelve weekly exercise sessions. Fewer people in the yoga group used pain-relief medication, too.

Although the researchers did not collect data to determine why yoga was such an effective therapy, participant comments suggested a number of factors, according to Karen Sherman, PhD, a Group Health researcher and the lead author of the study. Based on participant comments, Sherman surmised the following:

- Increased awareness of their bodies could have led patients to better posture and ergonomic practices.
- Better posture and ergonomic practices could have led patients to actions and behaviors that were less irritating to the back.
- Stress reduction and relaxation could have been important factors.

Another study done at a residential integrative health center in Bangalore, South India, compared physical exercise to yoga for chronic low-back pain patients. Some participants underwent seven days of a residential intensive yoga program comprised of physical postures, breathing practices,

YOGA AS PREVENTIVE MEDICINE

Yoga student and construction contractor Brian Highberger, from Lake Forest Park, Washington, believes yoga prevents painful flare-ups of his low-back problem. For roughly five years, Highberger's low back went out every few months, leaving him in bed icing and heating his back, taking Advil, and receiving massages until he was able to be mobile again. Brian's back pain stems from an old athletic injury and seems to radiate from his L3 vertebra.

Since starting a regular yoga practice—he takes a class at his local health club three or four times a week—he has had only one moderately painful episode.

Before he started practicing yoga, his debilitating back pain would leave him out of action for seven to ten days; after he started practicing yoga, he was back to his normal activities and pain free within three days. "There is no question that yoga helps my back problem. My core is stronger and my back is more supple and flexible, allowing me better range of motion," says Highberger. "It must be done on a regular basis though. I took a break from yoga last fall and that is when I had my one flare-up. I am still careful about lifting and twisting, but I don't have that constant worry that my back might go out at anytime."

meditation, and sessions on philosophical yoga concepts. The other participants practiced physical exercises with a physiatrist and attended sessions on lifestyle change. The yoga participants had a significant reduction in pain-related disability compared to the individuals in the exercise group. While both groups gained spinal flexibility, the people in the yoga group had greater spinal flexibility than the exercise participants did.

Yoga studies usually focus on a short time period, looking at people who participate in classes for a few months. The health benefits of a longer yoga practice are not often studied. Still, it would follow that the health benefits would increase the longer a person practiced yoga.

How Yoga Helps the Low Back

The book *Yoga as Medicine,* by Timothy McCall, MD, describes forty specific ways a yoga practice can improve a person's health. Some of the reasons that point directly to improving low-back function are that yoga:

- Improves balance
- Increases flexibility
- Strengthens muscles
- Improves posture
- Improves joint health
- Releases unconscious muscle gripping
- Relieves pain
- Reduces weight
- Increases oxygen supply to the tissues
- Nourishes intervertebral disks

Yoga can also improve an individual's psychological health, which is often a contributing factor in back problems. Practicing yoga can reduce levels of stress hormones, lessen depression, and relax the nervous system. Of course, all of these healing benefits are intertwined. During yoga sessions, participants breathe more slowly and deeply, which in turn leads to a relaxation response in the body. An hour or more spent doing yoga also takes you out of your life and its immediate stresses, which can lift your mood and relax your body.

Yoga works to bring the body, mind, and spirit into balance, and some believe this is why yoga can promote healing in the body. During yoga practice, you are asked to be in the present moment, focusing on what is going on in both your body and mind. "We frequently neglect our bodies, but we really can't separate out our thinking life from our physical life," says Jennifer Keeler, a certified yoga teacher who runs Yoga Momma at the Phinney Yoga House in Seattle. "Yoga brings our whole self into connection again. It allows us to recognize when we are stressed and out of balance, how the stress is affecting our overall well-being. Then it provides tools to begin making changes in our actions, resulting in balance."

Yoga also helps people take charge of their own health care. The more you learn about how your body feels and how your mind works, the more you can figure out what therapies are best for your own medical issues.

Types of Yoga

If you suffer from low-back pain, it is important to choose a yoga style with care. There are numerous types of yoga, and some are more appropriate than others for patients with back pain. People with back pain probably should avoid the following yoga styles:

- Ashtanga, or Power yoga
- Bikram, or Hot yoga
- Vinyasa yoga
- Some yoga classes at a gym

The above yoga styles focus on more vigorous movement: participants move quickly between poses without time to make adaptations for back issues. Some gym classes might be appropriate for persons with back pain; look for gentle yoga classes or therapeutic back classes. Yoga styles more appropriate for individuals with low-back concerns include:

- Iyengar yoga
- Viniyoga yoga
- Kripalu yoga
- Phoenix Rising Yoga Therapy
- Anusara yoga
- Integral yoga

Often a studio is not aligned with one specific yoga style. Teachers may have studied several types of yoga. The name a teacher gives her studio is often a synthesis of all she has learned during various trainings and through years of teaching yoga.

If, during your search, you come across a yoga style you don't recognize, ask if this style is appropriate for someone suffering from low-back pain. You should be able to adapt poses to fit your body's needs and minimize the risk of injury, and the teacher should have experience working with people with back issues.

Finding a Yoga Instructor

Finding the right yoga teacher is as important as choosing an appropriate style of yoga. If you have back issues, look for a studio with gentle or beginner-level classes, or a class that focuses on back issues. Sometimes you can find healthy-back classes at your local hospital. Some practitioners obtain a Yoga Alliance Membership (see "Resources," at the end of this book). This national organization helps lead the yoga movement in the United States by setting standards, fostering integrity, providing resources, and upholding the teachings of yoga.

Make sure your yoga instructor is trained and certified. There are no federal regulations in place, but there might be local regulations in your state. Whatever yoga style a teacher trains in, she should have completed at least a 200-hour level of training. Often instructors have completed training in more than one style; this diversity and depth of knowledge can be beneficial to students.

Call or meet with a potential yoga teacher. Ask the teacher the following questions:

- What kind of experience do you have working with people with low-back pain?
- Do you know how to adapt poses for someone with back issues?
- What yoga training have you done?
- Have you attended training in therapeutic practices for people with spine problems?

If the teacher has never worked with people with back problems, or she doesn't have any training in yoga and the back, she might not be the right instructor for you. You should feel comfortable with the teacher, since you will want to talk with her about adapting a pose when it doesn't feel right, or chat before class if you are having a flare-up of pain.

The potential teacher should also ask you what you want out of a yoga class. The studio should have a variety of classes, and asking this question will help the teacher determine what class is the best fit for you. Before you pick a yoga class, think about what you hope to gain from your practice. Some classes or teachers will be more appropriate than others for your needs. Are you looking for quiet, reflective time? Do you want a class that includes meditation or chanting? Are you hoping yoga will help you de-stress and relax? Everyone is unique, but the instructor can help create a practice that works for you.

Yoga Class

Your yoga teacher should be able to meet you where you are, physically and mentally. This means that if you are suffering from back pain, it's a good idea to have a few individual sessions—just you and the teacher—before joining a class. Tell the instructor about your doctor's diagnosis, your symptoms, and how you feel as you hold yoga postures. The teacher can observe how your body is moving, help you modify poses, and determine what class is appropriate for you. Perhaps you need to practice yoga while sitting, or use blocks and straps for some poses, or avoid some moves altogether.

In this vein, sometimes people with back pain shouldn't keep their legs straight during poses. Bending your knees still gives you the appropriate feeling and stretch. When you join a class, the teacher can tell you what poses to avoid and what adaptations you need to make for other poses. More importantly, you'll learn more about yoga and what moves and modifications are appropriate for you.

When you do join a class, remember that what is happening on your mat is the most important aspect of your session. Maybe some students seem more flexible than you seem, or another person's pose looks different from yours. The point of yoga is not about being super flexible or holding a posture that looks just like the one portrayed in a book. "It doesn't matter how you look, it matters how you feel. Can you breathe in the pose and what happens in your mind?" asks yoga teacher Cathy Prescott. "The postures are about finding a balance between effort and ease. You should be working just enough and relaxed just enough."

When you do a yoga pose, you should feel a stretch and be able to breathe. Stop and move out of a posture if you feel pain beyond the normal feelings of a muscle stretch. If you experience any grinding motion, heat, or sharp pains, this is also your cue to stop and talk to the teacher. One particular pose might not be appropriate for your body, or you might need to adapt the pose by using props or by moving your body in a different way.

Setting Up a Home Yoga Practice

While taking a yoga class even just once a week is beneficial, practicing yoga more often is even better. Although a group class can create community and people can challenge one another in class, a daily home practice will reap the most benefits for someone with low-back issues. Yoga teachers who are versed in therapeutic yoga recommend that any student suffering from back problems set up a daily home practice.

If you are taking private classes with an instructor, she can help you set up a home practice. If you are currently in a group class, it's easiest to set up a home practice by having a one-on-one session with your teacher. Yoga teacher Cathy Prescott likes to help her students create three distinct practices, each fifteen to twenty minutes in length. These short sessions can be put together if a person feels like doing a longer session on a particular day.

Meeting with a teacher helps you learn the poses correctly, as well as figuring out what props you will need to use at home. Starting a home practice often means investing in yoga equipment, including blocks, straps, bolsters, or stools. Sometimes using a chair or pillow you already own will suffice, and a wall is often an excellent prop.

An instructor might recommend just two to three yoga postures to do every day. Doing each pose correctly, with attention focused on your body and mind, is often the most vital part of practice. When you are ready to change your daily practice, meet with your instructor again. For some that is after a month, while other people find changing their home practice every six months works for them.

PILATES

Pilates isn't an ancient art, but its origin story is compelling. Joseph Pilates, born in Germany in 1880, created his own fitness regimen to help himself overcome several childhood illnesses. He believed his mind led his body to healing, and that others could follow a similar path through his fitness regimen. While held as a prisoner during World War I, he taught exercises to the other prisoners. He leaned the prison bed box springs against the wall and attached slings to them. The prisoners did various stretches with the help of the beds and slings, which were the very first Pilates exercise machines.

In the late 1920s, Joseph Pilates immigrated to the United States. Along with his wife, Clara, he started an exercise gym in New York City. Many of his first devotees were professional dancers. Today, dancers worldwide use his methods to stay in shape and help recover from injury. After he died in 1967, people continued to teach his basic mind–body fitness regimen, and this became known as the Pilates Method.

Quality of Movement

Today's Pilates practices have evolved from Joseph's original teachings. Well-trained teachers combine new knowledge about anatomy and movement, making current exercises more beneficial for students. Pilates is an exercise system that emphasizes breathing, concentration, control, precision, centering, and flow. With this focus, students work on spinal and pelvic alignment and core strength while performing exercises.

Although it's a heady proposition to keep six attributes in mind while executing exercises, this simply means that Pilates is about being conscious about your movements. These are tools used to create precise movements. "Pilates is about quality of movement more than the quantity of repetitions. Beautifully executing three sets of an exercise with control, precision, and proper breathing is much more beneficial than executing fifty repetitions without that focus to detail," says Marjorie Thompson, lead instructor and program director of the Pacific Northwest Ballet's Pilates program, PNB-Conditioning. "Breathing properly is essential to executing exercises efficiently. This carries over in your day-to-day life."

How Pilates Helps Your Back

An acute back injury or a chronic back problem can stem from muscular imbalances. Although no one has perfect posture, postural alignment can play a role in lumbar spine pain as well. Pilates helps promote muscular balance by developing a person's core strength. Joseph's definition of the core (called the *powerhouse* by Pilates practitioners) includes the abdominal, pelvic floor, buttocks, hip, and lower back muscles. During a class, you strengthen these muscles, build muscular endurance, and learn how to initiate movement from this powerhouse. This helps support your spine, alleviating back pain and preventing flare-ups of pain.

Rumor has it that practicing Pilates makes people taller. This doesn't mean you grow taller. This idea has its basis in better postural traits learned through practice. Pilates also builds leaner and longer muscles. If you choose to lift weights and become a body builder, this adds bulk to your frame. Pilates has the opposite effect. "I think the changes [that make people seem taller] come from body awareness, core strength, and pelvic and spinal alignment that inevitably lead to better posture," says Thompson. "We do dozens of easy chores that can be done with a mind–body connection or not. If I choose to engage my abdominal muscles and not lock my knees when I am picking up a stack of books, I will be making a healthy choice for my body that will benefit me and protect my back and my knees from unnecessary stress."

This mindfulness and better postural alignment carries over in everyday life. Maybe you walk with your shoulders rounded and your low back tucked in an irritating position. Through a Pilates practice, you'll begin to walk with your shoulders back and relaxed, and your low back in a more comfortable position, correcting poor postural traits and eliminating its corresponding pain. You'll learn to initiate muscles before you do some movements: before you get into a squatting position for gardening work, you'll engage the muscles you need to do the movement correctly, without hurting your lumbar spine.

Chronic back pain patients or people recovering from an acute injury or surgery can work with a Pilates instructor as part of their rehabilitation. (As always, check with your doctor before starting a practice.) A study reported in the *Journal of Orthopaedic & Sports Physical Therapy* in 2009 showed that exercising on Pilate's equipment helped lower pain intensity and improved functional disability in people with nonspecific low-back pain. Half of the study participants took part in a four-week Pilates training regimen designed to stabilize the lumbar-pelvic region. The other participants received usual care, meaning they consulted with health-care professionals as necessary.

"The equipment can support your spine. You have resistance that you are pushing and pulling against to give you some feedback. It gives you information about your body," says Stott Pilates instructor trainer Kristi Quinn, of Bodycenter Studios in Seattle.

Not all Pilates classes feature work on machines. Some classes use only mats—participants practice Pilates on exercise mats, using the effects of gravity. For someone with low-back pain, this might be difficult. Try a machine class or one-on-one machine sessions first, and ask the instructor if or when you might be ready for a mat class.

Finding a Pilates Instructor

As with yoga, there is not one unified Pilates-instructor certification process in the United States. When you check out a studio, it is important to ask if the instructors have undergone a training and certification process. There are numerous teacher-training programs, all with their own interpretations of Joseph Pilates's original regimen. If you are using Pilates as a rehab tool, find a practitioner trained in spinal rehabilitation and with experience in working with people with low-back pain issues. Ask the potential instructor the following questions about his certification process:

- How many hours of training were involved in actual practice? If he has trained for 900 hours, a majority if his training should be from doing Pilates as opposed to listening to someone talk.
- Did his training address back-pain issues, or does he have advanced training in working with low-back pain issues?
- Did he learn anatomy and how do to postural assessments on his students?

One way to find a reputable studio is to call your local professional dance company and ask where the dancers practice Pilates. There are studio and instructor locators on the Internet as well. Stott Pilates training programs include training in spinal rehabilitation. The Balanced Body Pilates website includes various types of Pilates studios. (For more information, see "Resources," at the back of this book).

Most Pilates studios have new students take one-on-one classes with an instructor. Each studio has its own rules concerning the number of individual classes students must take before they join a class setting. Executing a Pilates' movement correctly involves breathing correctly, tensing the right muscles, and moving in a controlled manner. You can practice Pilates without paying attention to these specifics, but your practice will lack the mind–body benefits, and some of the physical benefits. When you have ongoing back issues, it's vital to move with a teacher's input guiding you. The teacher should be checking your postural alignment, asking you how you feel as you move, and paying close attention to how you move. If you are there for a lumbar spine problem, expect the teacher to send you home with exercises to do every day. When your teacher feels you are ready for a group class, she will be able to direct you to the appropriate one.

If you are taking a regular Pilates class, set up a home practice by meeting privately with an instructor. If you buy home equipment, he can help you set it up and create an exercise regimen with you. As with at-home yoga practice, creating three fifteen to twenty minute daily practices will help keep your routine interesting and allow you to put the practices together for a longer at-home session. See your instructor again when you are ready for a new routine.

THE FELDENKRAIS METHOD

Your lumbar spine issues might be resolved through learning new postural and movement habits. The Feldenkrais Method is a movement education program that aims to ease chronic pain and tension and prevent acute pain flare-ups. Learning this system of gentle movements can improve your flexibility, balance, coordination, and posture.

Dr. Moshe Feldenkrais (1904–1984) developed the Feldenkrais Method after suffering from recurring knee injuries. Through his own self-awareness movement program, he was able to rehabilitate his knee. He was more interested in how well someone moved than in how perfectly he or she could sit or stand. Dr. Feldenkrais coined the term *acture* to reflect this idea. Optimal acture is the ability to move in any direction without preparation. When a Feldenkrais practitioner looks at someone sitting or standing, the practitioner evaluates how those patterns likely reflect the ways the person performs daily or recreational activities.

TAI CHI

If you go to any park in China or Southeast Asia, chances are you will see hundreds of people of all ages practicing the graceful, dance-like movements of *tai chi*. Also known as *tai qi* or *tai chi chu'an*, this ancient art form has been practiced in China for thousands of years. Tai chi is both a martial art and a health-promoting mind–body exercise regimen. The hundreds of movements that comprise this practice lessen stress by encouraging deep, slow breathing; improving flexibility and circula-tion; and building strength in the lower legs and hips. Tai chi can also be used as an adjunct therapy for people suffering from back pain. Practicing tai chi on a regular basis can improve body alignment, help-ing the back become more supple and fluent, which can lessen pain.

There are many tai chi styles. Some are practiced quite slowly while other forms have partici-pants moving fast and vigorously. To pick a class that fits your needs, observe or try a few different types of classes.

Picture a Barbie doll. She can't move well because her trunk is immobile. While other types of therapists might focus on helping Barbie achieve core strength, a Feldenkrais practitioner would help Barbie integrate her arm and leg movements with the movements of her midsection. Barbie's large muscles, joints, and small muscles should work cooperatively together. A Feldenkrais practitioner can help you identify your own habits of posture and movement, teaching you how to move in a more efficient and effective way.

If you see a Feldenkrais teacher for a one-on-one session—this is called a Functional Integration session—she will evaluate your postures and your movement patterns, assessing how these habits contribute to or even keep you in pain. She would choose hands-on techniques and exercises to help reduce symptoms. If you see a practitioner while you are having an acute flare-up of lumbar spine pain, she will place you in a comfortable posture that supports the back and helps turn off the spasms. Working with your breath while you are in a posture will help your body become more relaxed; this also alleviates pain.

Even if your pain isn't 100 percent relieved through the Feldenkrais Method sessions, you will learn how to move smarter, be aware of the habits that cause pain, and gain self-care skills. You can also join group sessions, called Awareness Through Movement classes. During a class, if a movement doesn't feel good, make the movement smaller, or do it in your imagination. Even imagining the movement can help train your body to do the movement, since brain messages precede actions.

A reputable practitioner completes a Guild Accredited Training Program—this takes roughly three to four years—through the Feldenkrais Guild of North America (see "Resources" at the back of this book).

THE ALEXANDER TECHNIQUE

Like the Feldenkrais Method, the Alexander Technique (AT) is based on the idea that physical problems are linked to your posture and body movements. In the 1890s, Australian Shakespearean actor Frederick M. Alexander created this method to cure his performance-linked laryngitis. Improving his head and neck posture put an end to his recurring ailment.

This movement therapy focuses on how the head sits on the body; this is called *primary control*.

If you see an Alexander Technique practitioner to help relieve your low-back pain, she will use hands-on coaching and exercises to help you learn more optimal ways of sitting, standing, and moving. Although this is a popular movement therapy for actors and musicians, research also shows benefits for people with back pain. Patients with back pain who took twenty-four AT sessions improved their ability to participate in activities by 42 percent, according to a study published in 2008 by the *British Medical Journal*. After one year, the AT group experienced back pain an average of three days a month, while the patients not learning AT typically experienced twenty-one days of back pain a month.

You can study the Alexander Technique in a group class or in one-on-one sessions with a teacher. Your practitioner will examine your posture in various positions, watch how you move, and take note of your breathing patterns. As you learn how to move in ways that ease tensions, the practitioner might guide you with his hands. Learning AT will take varying amounts of time for each student, but ten sessions are often recommended. Find a practitioner who is registered with the American Society for the Alexander Technique; to qualify, they must have trained for at least three years, undergoing a minimum of 1600 training hours (see "Resources" for more information).

6 PRACTICES FOR THE MIND

AS DISCUSSED IN CHAPTER 2, "The Mind–Body Connection," back pain is intrinsically connected with our minds, our emotions, and the stories we tell ourselves about a particular injury or pain experience. The hurt itself stems from a physical problem, but the pain signals sent to the brain become mixed up with other confusing messages, such as emotional reactions, justifications, denials, or condemnations—all the mental, emotional, and physiological reactions we have about pain.

The experience becomes not only about the physical hurt, but also about one's response to that hurt. What we think about an injury has the power to either lower or raise the level of pain we experience.

With chronic pain—even without changing the level of physical pain—you can make a tremendous positive impact on your symptoms by simply changing your reaction to the pain and creating a more positive story about the pain and your life. Doing this can lower the amount of pain you feel, lower your medication usage, and improve your quality of life. The story you tell yourself can affect your acute injury as well. The pain is real, but the way you react to it and the tales you create about the pain can either help heal an acute injury or help turn it into chronic low-back pain.

Practicing meditation can help bring relief to acute, subacute, or chronic low-back pain. Studies abound on the benefits of meditation. According to various reviews, meditation can help lessen anxiety, mild and moderate depression, excessive anger and hostility, insomnia, and high blood pressure; it can also prevent heart attacks and ease the symptoms of PMS, menopause, and arthritis.

People suffering from chronic back pain have also taken part in meditation studies. Mindfulness meditation had numerous benefits for the chronic back pain patients who took part in an eight-week study reported in *Pain* in 2008. (*Mindfulness* is one type of meditation practice.) These patients experienced less pain, improved physical function and pain acceptance, and better sleep.

Another study, reported in *NeuroReport* in 2006, showed that people skilled at meditation had a 40 to 50 percent lower brain response to pain than people who did not practice meditation. The people in this study practiced *transcendental meditation* (a mantra-based meditation practice). After the initial research was gathered, the nonmeditating participants learned transcendental meditation. Five months later, these twelve participants were retested. Now that they practiced meditation, their brain responses to pain had also dropped by 40 to 50 percent.

People with chronic low-back pain also found relief by practicing *breath therapy*, which blends breathing, meditation, and movement. A study done at the Osher Center for Integrative Medicine in San Francisco compared physical therapy to breath therapy for chronic low-back pain patients. After

YOGIC BREATHING

You can change your mood with your breathing. Try this exercise. First, think about how you feel at this moment. Now take five deep breaths in a row, while focusing on your breath. How do you feel now? Our breathing becomes shallow and short when we are nervous or in pain. By simply stopping and breathing deeply, you can influence your emotions, lessen fear and pain, and relieve stress. Yogic breathing, also called *diaphragmatic breathing*, is a simple relaxation exercise that everyone can learn:

- Put your hands on your stomach. Imagine that your belly is an inflatable mattress.
- Blow all your air out while imagining that the mattress is deflating. Your belly will shrink in.
- Then, take a deep breath in, and feel the mattress—your belly—inflate.

Most people only breathe from the chest up. Yogic breathing forces you to take a deeper breath, so you relax more effectively. One of the simplest, easiest ways to relax is to do ten of these breaths in a row.

six weeks, patients in both groups had less pain and had improved function. The people who practiced breath therapy also had improved coping skills and new insight into the effect of stress on the body.

WHAT IS MEDITATION?

Practicing meditation evokes the relaxation response, which lowers metabolism, blood pressure, heart rate, and breathing rates. Essentially, while you meditate, you calm your mind and slow down your body, creating balance and a sense of wholeness.

During meditation, you relax your logical mind, and then you access the part of the brain that is driving your subconscious. The subconscious is what you are acting from when you automatically respond to a painful fall from your bike or when you yell at your arguing children. You can think of meditation as giving your conscious self a nap, so you can talk positively to the subconscious mind. The way you talk to your subconscious depends on what type of meditation you practice. For example, with guided imagery, you envision what you want to happen. Some types of meditation use an affirmation or mantra to program your mind with positive thought. Meditation that involves movement might have you focus on a positive intention while you move.

By focusing on your breath and body, you place yourself in the present moment. This breaks the train of everyday thought, putting aside the past and the future. This momentary lapse from your life—whether it's ten minutes once a day or twenty minutes twice a day—has the power to help you rest deeply and feel better. Meditating is a skill you can learn that helps you focus on positive thought and on what you want to happen in life.

STRESS AND THE BODY

Think about how you respond to a stressful situation. Thanks to your lumbar spine pain, you have a hard time getting ready for work. The extra minutes it takes to get out of bed, put on clothes, make your breakfast, and walk your dog around the block have already put you behind schedule. Your low back's muscles, ligaments, tendons, and connective tissue—which are already hurting—tense up even more.

Then you encounter horrendous traffic on your way to work. You react immediately, without thinking: your body tenses even more, and your low-back pain intensifies, turning from a dull throb to radiating pain with shooting stabs of hurt. You curse out loud and your shoulders are so tight they almost touch your ears.

When faced with stress, your body responds via a built-in fight-or-flight mechanism (see Chapter 2 for an explanation of this mechanism). Your metabolism, blood pressure, heart rate, rate of breathing, and blood flow to the muscles increase.

"We secrete stress hormones, but we neither run nor fight," says Dr. Herbert Benson, director emeritus of the Benson-Henry Institute for Mind Body Medicine at Massachusetts General Hospital, and author of *The Relaxation Response*. "Stress is related to over 60 percent of visits to the doctor. No drugs or surgeries effectively treat this. Fortunately, just as we possess the fight-or-flight response, we as humans also have within us what's called the relaxation response. It is the biochemical, physiological, and genetic opposite of the fight-or-flight response."

Most of us don't realize we actually have a split second to think about how to respond to our stress. Usually we automatically behave based on how we have reacted in the past, according to the patterns we learned long ago. In that moment, we are actually at a place of choice. We can decide how to react. Meditation is a way of training the mind to recognize that moment, so we can respond in a way that is less stressful and more empowering.

MEDITATION BY ANY OTHER NAME

Meditation can be any type of activity that elicits the relaxation response in a person. Dr. Herbert Benson, one of the first doctors who connected meditation and Western medicine in the United States, coined the term *relaxation response* in the 1970s. He notes that all humans have the ability to evoke this calming body response, and you can choose the technique that works best for you.

Dr. Benson defined one relaxation response method, but this is just one of many types of techniques. Usually a method involves repetition, such as a word, a sound, a prayer, a phrase, or movement. One technique isn't better than another technique. Other forms of meditation include transcendental meditation, mindfulness meditation, tai chi, repetitive prayer, and walking meditation.

Practicing any movement therapy that has you focus on your breathing while moving your body with intention can be a meditative experience, including yoga, Pilates, or physical therapy exercises performed with meditative focus. If you have trouble sitting still, try yoga, tai chi, or walking meditation. If you like quiet, learn transcendental or mindfulness meditation.

With meditation, daily practice is the key. Practicing once a day is better than not practicing at all, meditating ten minutes twice a day is better still, and twenty minutes twice a day is the ideal.

The Relaxation Response Technique

The relaxation response method is easy to learn. Before you try it, pick a word or phrase to use during practice. This word, thought of as an affirmation, should be positive. If your word or phrase has a sacred component, it's called a mantra. Remember this means the word is sacred to you as an individual. Using a mantra can elevate a meditation practice, because the word is even more positive than an affirmation. Essentially, this word is programming your subconscious mind with positive thoughts. Examples of affirmations and mantras include "one" and "peace."

Now that you have your word, find a quiet place and sit down in a comfortable position. Close your eyes and focus on relaxing the muscles in your body. If this is hard for you, try starting at your toes and relaxing your body part by part. Then focus on your breathing. Breathe in slowly. As you breathe out, say your affirmation or mantra. Let's use the word *peace* as an example. Breathe in. Exhale while saying, "Peace." Continue doing this for ten to twenty minutes.

If you become distracted and other thoughts enter your mind, simply say, "Oh, well." Then return to your repetition, breathing in, and then exhaling while saying, "Peace." When you are done, open your eyes and sit for another minute or two. Practice the relaxation response twice a day. That's all there is to this simple method.

If Dr. Benson were leading the relaxation response for you, he might count your breaths at the beginning and end of your practice. Usually your breath rate would slow by a handful of breaths or more, proving the relaxing effects of this technique.

MASTERING MINDFULNESS AND EASING PAIN

Keep in mind that learning any form of meditation takes time, even movement therapies such as yoga or tai chi. You might give up too soon, not realizing this skill requires persistence.

Meditation is weight training for the mind. Think about preparing for a physical endeavor. You plan on climbing Mount Rainier or hiking twenty miles of the Appalachian Trail. You begin hiking smaller amounts every weekend, taking daily walks, and lifting weights at the gym. You cross-train by practicing other sports, you eat healthy foods, and you make sure to get plenty of sleep.

You couldn't summit Mount Rainier or complete your Appalachian hike without plenty of preparation. The mind works the same way. The first time you practice meditation, you won't automatically master it. Learning how to meditate takes practice, persistence, and discipline.

If you practice a form of meditation on a daily basis, you start to bring that frame of mind to your entire life. A strong meditation practice can help you recognize the moment where you get to decide how to react. When you feel your back ache as soon as you try to get out of bed in the morning, you can decide how to react. You can take five deep breaths, and respond with calmness. Instead of thinking how your whole day will surely be horrible now, you can think of strategies that will help you feel better or how you can arrange your day to work around the pain. You might lessen your pain through your deep breathing and intention to stay calm. At the very least, you might react more calmly to the situation, decreasing stress so you can avoid tensing up your muscles, which is a leading contributor to your back pain.

Transcendental Meditation

Dr. Benson studied transcendental meditation for his original research on the relaxation response. He realized that transcendental meditation, like many other meditative practices, elicited the relaxation response. There are numerous studies on the benefits of this form of meditation for anxiety, depression, and pain. To learn more about this technique, visit the Transcendental Meditation Program's website (see "Resources" at the back of this book). Learning transcendental meditation involves a seven-step course taught by a certified teacher. Go to the Transcendental Meditation Program's website to find a class near you.

A Mindfulness Practice

Mindfulness meditation stems from the Buddhist meditation tradition. Dr. Jon Kabat-Zinn began teaching Mindfulness-Based Stress Reduction (MBSR) when he founded the University of Massachusetts's Stress Reduction Clinic in 1979. The goal of mindfulness is to cultivate awareness of the present moment.

Eight-week MBSR classes are now taught at the Center for Mindfulness in Medicine, Health Care, and Society, an outgrowth of the original clinic, and at more than four hundred locales around the world (see "Resources" for more information). You can learn mindfulness meditation on your own. Unlike the relaxation response, mindfulness doesn't use an affirmation or mantra. Participants focus only on the breath. To practice mindfulness, find a quiet spot. Then:

- Sit in a straight-backed chair with your feet flat on the floor, or sit on the floor.

- Relax. You can do this by focusing on relaxing the muscles in your body, from your feet to the top of your head.
- Focus on your breathing—on the flow of air around your nostrils, on the feeling of the breath as it goes in and out, and on your belly as it rises and falls according to your breathing.
- If your mind becomes distracted, just come back to focusing on your breaths.
- Keep focusing on your breaths for twenty minutes.

By practicing mindfulness—or any type of meditation—for twenty minutes, twice a day, you are learning how to be aware of the present moment and learning how to focus your mind. With these skills, you can begin to be aware of that moment in time where you get to choose how to respond to an event in your life, such as that traffic jam on your way to work. If you usually react to a bout of back pain by getting angry and thinking your whole life is terrible due to your low-back pain, you can meditate with the intention to change this reaction. Next time you feel that familiar pain, you can focus on breathing deeply and staying calm. You can say to yourself, "Yes, my back hurts, and this is horrible right now. Still, in general, my life is good. How can I lessen my pain and still enjoy the rest of the day?" Meditation is training the mind to be in the present moment, both during practice and in your daily life.

Guided Imagery or Visualization

If you have never meditated, guided imagery or visualization is an easy-to-learn meditation style. You'll use your imagination to visualize a positive outcome. To practice:

MUSIC THERAPY

Listening to music can evoke the relaxation response. After composer, musician, and meditation practitioner David Ison broke his back, he created an acoustic therapy program to help himself walk again. Now called the TheraSound Method, a study published by the National Institutes of Health in 1999 documents this music program's ability to elicit the relaxation response. The participants—272 patients suffering from chronic pain problems—lowered their pain an average of 54 percent through this method.

After Ison injured his back, he noticed that meditation brought a reduction in pain and improved his concentration, which helped foster his healing. The music he created for TheraSound replicated the breathing pattern of meditation. People who listen to these compositions breathe in time to the music, which evokes the relaxation response in their minds and bodies.

While you can simply listen to TheraSound music as a form of therapy, you can also listen to these compositions while practicing other forms of meditation, using the sounds to help develop your practice. You can purchase acoustic therapy music by contacting TheraSound (see "Resources").

- Sit comfortably.
- Relax your body. You can do this by focusing on relaxing the muscles in your body, from your feet to the top of your head.
- Relax your conscious mind by focusing on your breathing for a while.
- Imagine a positive outcome for your ailment or problem. For back pain, you could imagine light going into your back and healing it. For changing how you react to traffic jams, focus your intention on changing your reaction to the inconveniences of modern life. Think of solutions for responding to the traffic jam while you meditate: breathing deeply; listening to soothing music; and realizing that your commute time is out of your control. You can focus your intention on ways to react to bouts of back pain as well, which might very well include the same tools as responding to the traffic jam.
- Practice this twice a day for twenty minutes.

You can purchase guided imagery and visualization tapes, CDs, and DVDs. These can be helpful tools if you are new to meditation, or if you are looking for structured guidance. The Benson-Henry Institute offers guided relaxation CDs online, along with relaxation response method CDs (turn to "Resources"). Some yoga classes have a guided imagery component. You can also look for guided imagery and visualization classes in your community.

Walking As Meditation

If you like to move, walking meditation might be a good fit for your lifestyle. If you cannot remember the last time you sat still, try this method. Mindfulness guru Dr. Kabat-Zinn has his students walk in circles in a room or back and forth in a lane while learning walking meditation. To practice

walking meditation, follow tips culled from Dr. Kabat-Zinn's book *Full Catastrophe Living: Using the Wisdom of Your Body and Mind to Face Stress,
Pain, and Illness*:

- While walking, focus on sensations in one part of your body. Beginners
  can focus on just their feet, or just their legs. Be aware of each foot or
  leg as it moves.
- Add in an awareness of your breathing as you walk.
- If you lose focus and your mind wanders, just bring your attention back
  to each foot or leg as it moves, and again focus on your breathing.
- Focus your gaze in front of you instead of looking at your feet or at the
  sights around you.
- You can walk at any pace, slow or quick.
- Practicing walking meditation alone is a way to be less self-conscious
  about learning it, and can help with focus.
- While you are learning walking meditation, practice it for short peri-
  ods, perhaps five or ten minutes.

As you become an adept meditative walker, you won't need to walk in
circles or back and forth from wall to wall. You can practice walking meditation for longer periods of time, maybe even for miles on an outside trail.
After you are adept at concentrating on just one body part, try focusing on
your whole body and its sensations.

PREPARING MENTALLY FOR SURGERY

Studies show that relaxation techniques, positive thinking, and guided imagery and visualization practices not only help you prepare for back surgery and post-operative recovery, but also increase your chances of a successful outcome and a faster recovery. One program that has proven particularly effective was developed by psychotherapist Peggy Huddleston and is described in her book *Prepare for Surgery, Heal Faster: A Guide of Mind–Body Techniques*. Huddleston, a psychotherapist, recommends the following five steps as a means of preparing for surgery. Her book and the accompanying CD (or tape or MP3 file) guide you through each of these steps.

- Relax to feel peaceful.
- Visualize your healing.
- Organize a support group.
- Use healing statements.
- Establish a supportive doctor-patient relationship.

Forty-four people who both took part in Huddleston's workshop and used her techniques before and after knee replacement surgery had less anxiety on the day of their operation, and left the hospital 1.3 days sooner than patients who did not use these techniques or attend the workshop, according to an unpublished study on Huddleston's website (see Resources). Huddleston's procedures can also be used to make your post-operative recovery process easier, faster, and more successful.

"Mind–Body Surgery Preparation" in Chapter 9 describes in detail Huddleston's steps and materials; please turn to those pages for complete information.

7 BODYWORKS

HANDS-ON THERAPIES CAN BE INCREDIBLY HEALING. Called *bodyworks*, these modalities are numerous and varied. A bodywork therapy might be an integral part of your care plan. Adding one or more of these complementary practices to your medical care might promote healing, ease pain, and contribute to a sense of wholeness.

Sometimes it is hard to imagine how bodyworks fit into medical care. Perhaps you haven't heard of some of the therapies discussed in this chapter. Not all of these practices are understandable in Western medical terms. Some techniques focus on meridians, invisible energy channels that you will not find in a Western-style anatomical drawing. This doesn't mean such techniques won't be beneficial for your specific low-back issue.

Think of the wheel of medical care options we've talked about throughout this book—the spokes represent the plethora of health-care options, including bodyworks. Stepping onto the hub, you are in charge of your medical care, gathering information and working with knowledgeable practitioners who listen and see you as a whole person. What bodyworks therapies might help alleviate or even prevent future episodes of lumbar spine pain?

Sometimes a practice won't be the right fit for you or for your low-back problem. If you try a bodyworks therapy and don't find any relief or see any progress after a handful of sessions, it might be time to move on. This can be discouraging. Still, it's worthwhile to try new paths to healing, whether that means trying a different bodywork technique or talking to your back specialist about other options.

It's also helpful to think about the term *healing*, which isn't defined by a cure. "*Healing* implies the possibility for us to relate differently to illness ... as we learn to see with eyes of wholeness," writes Jon Kabat-Zinn, PhD, in *Full Catastrophe Living*. There isn't always a complete cure for low-back pain, but you can begin to see yourself as a whole person with low-back pain. Healing might mean learning self-care methods to alleviate your pain, seeing a bodyworks practitioner and your doctor as needed, and living your daily life as fully as possible. Your path to healing is a unique journey. Read on to learn more about bodyworks therapies.

MASSAGE

Massage is an ancient, manual hands-on therapy, although a practitioner might apply pressure to your body not only with his hands, but also with his elbows, forearms, knees, or feet. Hippocrates, often called the father of medicine, wrote this in 460 BC: "The physician must be experienced in many things, but assuredly in rubbing."

Today, more than eighty types of therapies fall within the category of *massage*. These manual therapies treat the body's muscles, ligaments, joints, skin, and connective tissues. Various types of massage attempt to affect whole systems of the body, including the lymph nodes and the gastrointestinal, musculoskeletal, circulatory, and nervous systems. At the very least, people with low-back pain have some level of muscle tightness or guarding happening in their bodies. Massage helps relax the body.

Patients with persistent back pain found massage to be an effective tool for relieving symptoms and increasing function, according to a review of studies published in 2003 by the Group Health Research Institute. This systematic review of studies also concluded that massage therapy might reduce the costs of care after an initial course of therapy for back pain. Massage can be a holistic therapy, treating the mind, body, and spirit. The human connection inherent in massage fosters a sense of well-being and wholeness.

Choosing a Massage Style or Therapist

How do you find the type of massage that is right for you and your specific condition? Picking a type of massage is similar to picking a yoga style. The yoga style you choose is dependent on the expertise of the teacher leading the class. "Any system of massage that lasts long enough to be well-known is likely to have value, but that value is only as good as it is artfully applied by the practitioner," says Wolfgang Brolley, a massage therapist and physical therapist who practices in Seattle.

Any practitioner whom you see for your low-back pain problem is likely to have massage-therapist recommendations. Ask friends and family if they have received an excellent massage from a local therapist. It's not as easy to find a massage practitioner by looking online, but it can be a good starting place. The National Certification Board for Therapeutic Massage

& Bodywork (NCBTMB) certifies massage and bodywork practitioners (see "Resources," at the back of this book). To receive this accreditation, a therapist must show mastery of a core skill set, pass an exam, uphold the NCBTMB's standards of practice and code of ethics, and take part in continuing education programs. Currently, forty-three states regulate massage therapists, and several states have pending legislation. Ask your potential therapist if he or she has accreditation through your state or a local governing board.

Obviously, a lengthy discussion of every style of massage would merit a book of its own. We'll discuss several types of massage. Most of the bodyworks practices in this chapter also fall within the massage category. For a more thorough list of styles with accompanying descriptions, look online at "Massage Today," a web-based massage therapy publication (turn to "Resources").

When you imagine a massage, you are probably picturing *Swedish massage.* Known as classic massage in Sweden and parts of Europe, this style originated during the eighteenth century in Sweden. Considered the most common massage type, Swedish massage incorporates five basic strokes— long gliding strokes, kneading, striking or tapping, vibration or shaking, and rubbing—to work the muscles and connective tissue. This relaxing style of massage lessens pain, improves circulation and range of motion, and helps to detoxify the body's tissues. When your body's muscles are tense, chemical waste products stagnate, causing irritation and pain; Swedish massage helps eliminate this waste. Swedish massage is the underlying technique for several other massage styles. *Deep tissue massage* focuses on loosening up the deepest muscle layers. *Sports massage* uses techniques from both Swedish and deep tissue massage to prevent injury and to aid in healing after injury occurs. Athletes also use sports massage to keep their bodies in optimal condition for competition.

Therapeutic Massage from A to Z

We won't cover every letter in the alphabet, but the following types of therapeutic massage might relieve your low-back pain.

Acupressure therapists focus pressure on the anatomical points used in acupuncture. Instead of needles, therapists use their hands to restore flow to invisible energy channels called meridians. For more information on this massage style, see this chapter's "Acupuncture" section.

CranioSacral therapy (CST) works with the membranes that surround the brain and spinal cord, called *dura mater*. According to CST therapists, these membranes have a slow but palpable motion or pulse; CST therapists can feel this pulse throughout the body. Disturbances or blocks in this pulse negatively affect your nervous system. A CST practitioner restores this pulse.

Physical therapists often use *myofascial release* techniques on patients. Fascia are the connective tissues that envelop the entire body. If you removed all the other matter in the body, this spider web of tissues would still create the structure of your body. Myofascial release finds the areas of your body where the fascia is stuck, scarred, or immobile. The therapist applies slow and steady pressure to these tissues, promoting healing.

Reflexology operates from the principle that reflex points on the hands and feet correspond to points on the rest of the body. Reflexologists use massage and pressure on the hands and feet to encourage healing at various places in the body. Some practitioners also work on a patient's ears.

Shiatsu technically means *finger pressure*. During this Japanese massage style, the therapist uses massage techniques on the invisible energy channels, or meridians, of your body, as opposed to using needles as in acupuncture. Practitioners may use their thumbs, fingers, palms, and feet to massage you.

Dating back more than 2000 years, *Thai massage* actually had its beginning in India. Depending on training, therapists use a combination of gentle massage, acupressure, stretching, and placing patients in positions similar to yoga poses.

Trigger points are painful areas, bands, or knots in muscles. In the 1940s, Dr. Janet Travell mapped the body's trigger points. During *myofascial trigger-point therapy*, a practitioner locates the trigger points that need release, uses pressure to relieve the point, and usually massages the area after this release.

Stemming from Chinese medicine principles that date back centuries, *tuina* (*twee nah*) aims to restore flow in blocked or stagnant energy channels. During a treatment, the practitioner applies massage techniques on anatomical points, meridians, muscles, and nerves.

A French osteopath pioneered *visceral manipulation*. *Viscera* means organs, and this type of massage focuses on imbalances between your organs and corresponding body structures. For example, pain that shoots down the front of the leg can be a referred pain from one of your organs.

THE BOWEN TECHNIQUE

Created by Australian Thomas Bowen in the 1950s, this soft-tissue technique has several monikers, including Bowenwork, Bowen therapy, and Bowen Technique. A Bowen therapist uses a stretch-and-roll-through technique. By stretching a tissue, she challenges the tissue for a brief moment, then she moves over that point in a perpendicular fashion and creates a muscular release, as well as sending a neurologic message to the brain that helps the body recharge. Bowen believed the body has a natural ability to heal itself, and that his technique helped the body reset itself.

During a Bowen session the therapist will actually leave the room from time to time, giving each body section a few minutes to begin responding to the moves. The Bowen Technique works in a sequential way to help the whole system. Therapists believe Bowenwork returns the body to a state of homeostasis.

If you see a Bowen therapist for a low-back problem, whether it is acute or chronic, she will do a physical assessment, checking your posture and looking for muscular and connective tissue restrictions anywhere in your body. The therapist will work to release the tension in the primary site of pain and also address other issues throughout the entire body. Although the number of sessions varies, you can expect marked improvement after three or four treatments. Many Bowen Technique patients say they feel an overall sense of well-being from these therapeutic sessions. If you have chronic low-back pain or compensatory postural positions have developed over the years, a longer period of therapy may be necessary.

ROLFING

Rolfing has a beginning similar to countless other therapies and exercise regimens. Ida Rolf created this soft-tissue manipulation and movement education program because she was seeking solutions for her and her sons' medical ailments. (One unique story feature: Ida Rolf earned her PhD in biochemistry in 1920, the same year women in the United States were granted the right to vote.)

Dr. Rolf coined the term *Structural Integration* for her deep-tissue massage therapy program. Today, people commonly call her technique *Rolfing*, although the formal name is "The Rolfing Technique of Structural Integration." Dr. Rolf believed that the connective tissue holds the body together and gives us our shape. Picture your connective tissue as a spider web linking all the body parts; this web would still hold your body's structure even if someone took out everything else in your body. Dr. Rolf believed that as we age, our connective tissue becomes misaligned, as well as less elastic and tough, placing demands on the rest of the body and causing poor postural traits. Rolfers use a variety of pressures to manipulate the fascia. This realigns the body structure within this connective tissue, helping to correct postural traits and balance the body within gravity.

If you see a Rolfer for your low-back pain, he might suggest undergoing what is called the *Ten Series,* a standardized recipe of Rolfing. A Ten Series practitioner will aim to systematically balance and optimize both the structure and movement of your entire body by the end of ten sessions. During your first visit, the practitioner will look at your body as you stand and as you move. Your Rolfer will apply pressure to your body with his fingers, knuckles, and elbows at the level where the connective tissue begins to release. This can be an intense experience, and Rolfing might feel painful at times. Rolfers believe the patterns that can cause pain in the body are not only physical, but emotional as well. Rolfing frees up both physical and emotional restrictions. You might cry, or laugh, or have other emotional reactions to this physical therapy. Sometimes practitioners recommend a form of psychological therapy to help with these issues. The time between sessions—sometimes weeks or even months—gives your body and mind time to process the therapy and integrate the physical, emotional, and psychological changes into your life.

Practitioners don't always prescribe the Ten Series; you might have a handful of visits or a dozen appointments. You might see a reduction or a complete alleviation of pain through this therapy. You can also expect to learn better postural traits and become more aware of your body. Rolfers are licensed through the Rolf Institute of Structural Integration (see "Resources" at the back of this book).

HELLERWORK STRUCTURAL INTEGRATION

Joseph Heller, the founder of Hellerwork, was actually the first president of Dr. Ida Rolf's Rolf Institute. Branching off from Dr. Rolf's work, Heller further addressed the spiritual and emotional aspects of the mind and body. Along with structural integration bodywork, Hellerwork includes movement-posture education and body-centered dialogue.

As with Rolfing and other forms of Structural Integration, a Hellerwork practitioner uses deep tissue massage to restructure your body's fascia. This releases tension, allowing changes in posture and movement patterns. Movement education is intrinsic in each session. You will learn new ways to sit, stand, and move through the practitioner's touch and guidance. The practitioner and client acknowledge and discuss ("dialogue about") the psychological issues that come up during a session. The dialogue component stems from the belief that our emotions manifest themselves in our bodies and their movements.

Hellerwork sessions explore the psychology of "selves," examining the idea that every person has multiple selves, or parts. Because of a person's personal history, certain aspects of a person's personality tend to come to the forefront, becoming a central aspect of how she lives her life, which then influences posture. Let's say the "pusher aspect" of a person's personality is strong; that is, she *pushes* to get everything done. This aspect of her personality isn't interested in relaxing in Hawaii. Hellerwork strives to help a person notice such dominant parts, or selves, as well as opening the patient up to other aspects of her personality. By bringing conscious awareness to your entire personality, Hellerwork aims to give you more choices, leading to a fuller life. Joseph Heller calls this the "coming home to your body" principle.

Your first visit to a Hellerwork practitioner will involve the same physical assessment used by other bodyworks practices: the practitioner will observe your body's structure, posture, and movement patterns. Hellerwork has an eleven-session series designed to realign the body systematically while releasing chronic tension and stress. For example, the first session focuses on the theme of inspiration. This session centers on the rib cage, breath, and what inspires you and fulfills your spirit. While these are the jumping-off points for a Hellerwork appointment, each patient and session is unique. Your practitioner might prescribe a different number of sessions based on your specific needs.

A certified Hellerwork practitioner has graduated from a Hellerwork International School, is licensed and insured, partakes in continuing education workshops, and follows a professional code of ethics and standards (see "Resources," at the back of the book).

Other Structural Integration Therapies

Besides Hellerwork, numerous other bodyworks therapies stem from Dr. Rolf's original work. These practices are based on the idea that gravity, everyday life, injuries, movement patterns, and attitude can affect your body structure, leading to pain. As in Rolfing and Hellerwork, practitioners in these other therapies use massage techniques to restructure the body's fascia and overall physical structure. Depending on the type of Structural Integration practice, a session may also include movement education;

emotions and behavior patterns may be assessed as well. Each type of Structural Integration practice looks to balance the whole person. You can find Structural Integration practitioners at the International Association of Structural Integration website (turn to "Resources"). This site includes links to several bodyworks organizations, such as the Soma Institute of Neuro-muscular Integration, the Institute of Structural Medicine, and Kinesis Myofascial Integration.

CHIROPRACTIC CARE

Chiropractic therapy works with the biomechanics of the backbone to re-store function to the body. The spine's top twenty-four vertebrae connect above and below, and each one of these connections can move in six dif-ferent ways. A lack of movement or flexibility in a joint can cause pressure on the joint and the surrounding tissues, perhaps irritating the nerve roots and putting nearby muscles into spasm. A chiropractor maneuvers and massages the spinal joints—a process called *spinal manipulation*—aiming to restore full mobility to the specific joints and the body.

"Chiropractic care is an art form on top of a diagnostic skill. You have to find the joint that is restricted or locked, and then use your hands-on skill to help the patient gain full function," says Lew Estabrook, a Seattle-area chiropractor. "Similar to a surgeon, the chiropractor has to have good diag-nostic skills with good techniques to get effective results. If one chiroprac-tor does not solve a health issue, do not give up. Try a second chiropractic opinion."

Finding a skilled chiropractor is important. Ask friends, family, and your other practitioners for referrals. A licensed chiropractor has done a minimum of two years of pre-med courses and then graduated from a four-year academic chiropractic program and passed state or national exams, earning a doctor of chiropractics, or DC, title.

During your first visit, the chiropractor will take a thorough history of your systemic problems, and you will undergo a movement-oriented examination. Some practitioners always take X-rays or other diagnostic images, while others order imaging only for some patients. During an adjustment or treatment, your practitioner will use a variety of hands-on techniques to put pressure on the joint or joints. Often literature on chiropractic care talks about a cracking or popping noise that signals repositioning. This is just one technique, and your practitioner might not use this style of care during a visit. Even if your chiropractor uses this high-velocity technique, your body might not have an audible response. The goal of treatment is to restore more normal function to the joint, taking pressure off the surrounding muscles, ligaments, and nerve tissue. This gives your body an opportunity to go through its normal healing process.

Every chiropractic patient has a unique schedule of appointments, but you should see some results after a handful of visits. As your body begins responding to treatment, often your chiropractor will have you do exercises and stretching to help restore strength and stamina to your back and body. Similarly, your chiropractor might recommend other types of care to help with your low-back pain issue. Some chiropractors might recommend adjustments on an ongoing basis, although no studies have shown a benefit for seeing a chiropractor for long-term treatment. Look for a practitioner who has a clear timeline for treatment, with an end in sight. A Group Health Research Institute review of evidence, reported in a 2003 issue of

Annals of Internal Medicine, found that spinal manipulation had roughly the same clinical benefits as conventional medical treatments, such as over-the-counter pain relievers and physical therapy.

OSTEOPATHY

Osteopathic doctors also practice spinal manipulation. American physician Andrew Taylor started osteopathy after concluding that the musculoskeletal system is fundamental to the health of the body. While osteopathic doctors have learned Western medical practices, they also have studied osteopathic manipulation and holistic health practices. While seeing an osteopath is similar to visiting an MD, treatments can also include:

- Osteopathic manipulation
- Physical therapy
- Movement and exercise education
- Nutrition
- Reducing stress through relaxation techniques

As opposed to chiropractic care, which tends to focus on manipulating the spinal column, osteopathic manipulation addresses the entire musculoskeletal system. Like other bodywork practices we have talked about, osteopathic medicine aims to put the entire body into balance: mind, body, and spirit. By seeing a doctor of osteopathy (a DO), you can seek both conventional treatments as well as a range of complementary therapies (listed above). To learn more about osteopathic medicine or to find a DO in your area, log onto the American Osteopathic Association website (find this information in "Resources," at the back of this book).

ACUPUNCTURE

It's safe to say that acupuncture is one of the oldest medical practices still used in the world today. The earliest known records state that acupuncture grew out of Wu Shamanism in the Shang Dynasty, with the first needles fashioned out of bone. As acupuncture has evolved over a 5,000-year period, it has been influenced by various cultures as well as by Taoist, Buddhist, and Confucian philosophies. While acupuncture has progressed and changed, the art remains rooted in traditional models and theories that have been tried and tested in clinical applications.

Acupuncture aims to restore the flow of *qi* in a patient's body. *Qi* (pronounced *chee*) is a living dynamic that, for lack of a better word, is often translated as "energy." In theory, the *qi* courses through the human body via pathways called *meridians* or *channels*. An obstruction (stagnation), excess, or deficiency of *qi*—due to trauma or changes in your body—can upset the balance of *qi* in your body. This produces physical discomfort that can manifest itself as pain, whether that pain is local or throughout an entire system in your body.

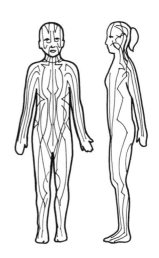

In 1997, the National Institute of Health delivered a Consensus Development Conference Statement in support of acupuncture. The statement said reasonable studies showed satisfactory results in patients using acupuncture as a treatment for low-back pain and myofascial pain.

7.1. Meridians or Channels

If you see an acupuncturist for your back pain, you will be treated for both the presenting symptom (pain) and the root cause of the imbalance. The acupuncturist may employ several traditional methods of examination to determine the root cause, including taking a complete medical history, a pulse diagnosis, abdominal diagnosis (called a *hara diagnosis*), facial diagnosis, tongue diagnosis, and also looking for signs of blood stagnation and swelling if there is back pain due to trauma. The acupuncturist should be conversant with Western medical protocol as well. After the exam, the practitioner will weave together a diagnosis based on what is presenting at the time.

As treatment begins, the practitioner selects pre-sterilized filiform needles made from stainless steel. The practitioner will insert the needles locally at the site of the injury, as well as distally along the channel pathways. Many people wonder how much acupuncture hurts. Often people say that the process is painless, or that the needles hurt less than yanking on a single strand of hair. The acupuncturist might also choose a form of heat therapy called *moxibustion,* in which the herb mugwort is either burned on the head of the needle or applied directly to the skin. This produces an increase in the flow of blood and *qi* systemically and locally in the body. Where there is stagnation of blood, the application of cups (a process called *cupping*) can be used to break up adhesions and old stagnation. As acupuncture is a hands-on form of medicine, bodywork and massage are also employed. Acupuncture naturally increases the circulation of blood, lymph, and *qi* in the body. This relieves your body of discomfort and allows your body to restore its own healing properties.

A course of acupuncture treatment usually takes between five to ten sessions, depending on the severity of the injury, how long the problem has been in the body, your age, and your constitution. Usually you will not need to get fully undressed, but simply roll up your sleeves and your pant legs. Sometimes you'll need to get undressed down to your underwear. Each session takes about an hour.

Some doctors are trained in acupuncture. There are different state requirements for doctors obtaining an acupuncture degree; you'll want to verify that your doctor holds a certified state license. Practitioners who aren't MDs obtain a masters degree in acupuncture and undergo a comprehensive accreditation procedure through the National Certification Commission for Acupuncture and Oriental Medicine (NCCAOM). Locate an acupuncturist online at the NCCAOM website, or by logging onto Acufinder.com, an online resource for acupuncture, Chinese herbs, and Asian medicine (see "Resources").

HYPNOTHERAPY

If you can recall the sensation of falling asleep, you are familiar with the state of hypnosis. Just as you start to drift off to sleep with your eyes closed, yet while you are still aware of sounds, feelings, and sensations, you are passing through a state of hypnosis. Similarly, when you wake in the morning, you are aware of the sounds of birds, the feeling of somatic sensations in your body, and although your eyes are still closed, you are aware of the room being lit by soft, morning light. Once again, you are coming through a state of hypnosis. We experience trance or hypnosis many times during the day. While you are in trance, your conscious mind steps aside, allowing the unconscious mind to step into the spotlight. An important note: all hypnosis is self-hypnosis. Even though the hypnotist is "inducing" the trance, the practitioner has no power or control over the subject.

Hypnosis has a long history in the field of pain management. The National Institute of Health has officially endorsed it as an effective treatment for pain alleviation. Hypnosis can also lower your heart rate and blood pressure, and lead to relaxation. If you need surgical intervention for your back problem, it's also an effective way to lessen pre-surgical anxiety and lower post-surgical pain and complications.

Seek a practitioner with experience in using hypnosis for pain management. During your appointment, the hypnotist will take a complete medical history. Then the practitioner will explain hypnosis with a pre-induction talk. The trance state develops through the building of rapport and various techniques. Helping you achieve a deep state of trance is accomplished in several ways, including progressive relaxation, eye fixation, eye opening and closing while counting backward, arm catalepsy, and confusion inductions.

Once you have achieved trance, the hypnotist uses techniques that involve various suggestions, images, and unconscious learnings to teach you how to be pain free, or, at the very least, how to control uncomfortable sensations in your body.

Although there is no national standard licensing system for hypnotists, the largest organization for health and mental health-care professionals using clinical hypnosis in the United States is the American Society of Clinical Hypnosis (ASCH). You can find a hypnotherapist on the ASCH website (turn to "Resources," at the back of this book).

8 FOODS, HERBS, AND SUPPLEMENTS

"YOU ARE WHAT YOU EAT" is a nice phrase, but what does it really mean? When you have low-back pain, is there a direct stomach–back connection? Maybe that candy bar you ate for a snack wasn't the best choice, but can it really intensify your lumbar spine pain?

Inflammation often causes pain and swelling. As explained in Chapter 2, "The Mind–Body Connection," if you cut your finger, it usually doesn't hurt very much at first. A day or so later, though, your cut and the somewhat swollen area around it feels worse. That's because your body's defense system, otherwise known as your immune system, started an inflammatory process to heal the cut. The chemicals sent to heal your injury are actually irritating the nerves around the cut.

Sometimes this inflammatory response is too strong, causing even more pain. Let's say your brain is sending chemicals to repair a slight tear in a back muscle due to a lumbar sprain-strain. This inflammatory-response team sends cells to the area to help it repair, but the chemicals the cells release can irritate the nerves, which causes more pain and increases muscle spasms. If the response is too vigorous and goes on too long, it can result in scarring, which makes the tissue less flexible and more prone to injury the next time you play basketball.

You can modulate your body's inflammatory process through diet, supplements, and herbs. Through simple changes, you can decrease your likelihood of generating an overly high inflammatory response. This might not only ease the pain caused by your low-back injury, but might also positively affect other health issues related to inflammation.

HOW DIET HELPS

You need your body's inflammatory-response system to live. Without it, even that simple finger cut wouldn't heal. Sometimes, however, the inflammatory-response system overreacts. Imagine dropping a wine bottle on the floor and watching it shatter. Instead of picking up the pieces yourself, you call a fire squad and a police team, along with a hundred friends to clean up the mess. All of these people end up creating a greater mess in your kitchen than any shattered wine bottle. In like manner, your inflammatory-response team can worsen a problem.

Through changing your diet, you can help regulate your inflammatory process. Several elements in the diet determine the level of your inflammatory response, including types of fat in your body, as well as the amount of antioxidants and phytochemicals available for your body to use.

Fatty acids are considered the building blocks of fats. Our bodies cannot make essential fatty acids. We obtain fatty acids from the food we eat. Fatty acids change the type of chemicals your body's immune system secretes during an inflammatory reaction. By changing the types of fats you consume, you can change the level of inflammation you experience. Two types of fats essential for our bodies are omega 6 and omega 3 fats. Most Americans consume too much omega 6 fat in comparison to omega 3 fat. This imbalance promotes inflammation in the body. You can decrease inflammation by increasing your intake of omega 3 fat to balance the ratio of omega 6 to omega 3.

Antioxidants are compounds found in foods, especially in fruits and vegetables, which quench the inflammatory response and protect tissues from damage by blocking free radicals. Free radicals are unstable compounds generated in the inflammatory process that can damage DNA and cells.

Phytochemicals are compounds found naturally in plants that have numerous health benefits, including anti-inflammatory ability. Examples of phytochemcials include flavinoids, which are often found in berries. Flavinoids may actually deactivate enzymes that promote inflammation.

Below are diet suggestions that can help regulate your immune system, so the next time your low-back pain flares up, there is less pain and swelling during the healing process and less chance of scar tissue forming in your body.

EAT THESE FOODS

Want to help decrease inflammation in your body (and in your poor aching back)? Here's a primer on types of food to include in your diet. Eating these healthy foods is an easy way to possibly lower your pain level and decrease your immune system response the next time you suffer a bout of low-back pain.

Cold-Water Fish

The acronym *SMASH* stands for salmon, mackerel, anchovies, sardines, and herring. Try to include these types of fish in your meal plan. SMASH is a good starting point for including fish in your diet, but eating all types of cold-water fish can have anti-inflammatory benefits.

Fruits and Vegetables

Increase your daily intake of fruits and vegetables. Although all fruits and vegetables have anti-inflammatory properties, try to include the ones with the darkest pigments. Berries—blueberries, raspberries, blackberries, strawberries—have the most benefits for your body. Likewise, the greenest vegetables are your best bet, such as broccoli, spinach, and winter greens. Deep-colored fruits and veggies have more plant pigments and vitamins per bite, which contain antioxidants. These substances can actually deactivate enzymes that promote inflammation.

Whole Grains and High-Fiber Foods

Add whole grains and high-fiber foods to your menu. Whole grains and high-fiber foods balance your insulin response. There is a relationship between your insulin response and your inflammation. When you eat sugar, a hormone called insulin increases. If you eat refined sugar, you get a larger insulin response in comparison to eating a small amount of sugar while also consuming a whole grain or high-fiber food. Having chronically high insulin levels is associated with increased inflammation.

When you are buying grains, look for the color brown. Choices include brown rice, whole grain breads, whole grain pastas, spelt, buckwheat, and barley. Learn how to cook these grains from whole foods or vegetarian cookbooks, such as *Vegetarian Cooking for Everyone* (see "Bibliography" at the end of this book). High-fiber foods include fruits, vegetables, and whole grains. Other examples include beans or legumes. Add any legume to your weekly menu: lentils, split peas, and garbanzo, red, pinto, and black beans.

Water
You have heard it before, but we will say it again: drink more water. Aim to drink eight glasses of H_2O every day.

AVOID THESE FOODS
Parallel to the list of foods to include in your diet are foods to decrease or avoid. The following foods can increase inflammation, leading to more pain. Minimize these food types in your menu plan.

Red Meat and High-Fat Dairy Products
Red meat and high-fat dairy products such as cheese and whole milk contain *saturated fat*—a type of fat that promotes inflammation. It is best to reduce your intake of saturated fats. If you still want to eat red meat, limit your intake and try to buy grass-fed meat, which is better for your body.

Sugar
Avoid refined sugar, including white sugar, brown sugar, and high-fructose corn syrup. All sugars impair the functioning of your immune system. Even sugar in its natural form—molasses, honey, and maple syrup—should not be a regular part of your diet.

White Foods
Take white foods off your recipe ingredient list. Try to remove white flour, white bread, and white rice from your pantry.

Flavored Drinks

Don't be swayed by flavored bottled waters. Take a pass on any flavored drinks, including soda pop, vitamin-style waters, lemonade, and juice. Avoid these sugar-laden drinks.

Processed Foods

Avoid processed foods. Buy whole foods, meaning products that have not undergone extensive manufacturing processes. Fruits, vegetables, and whole grains have had little done to them before they reach your local grocery store. Foods with ingredients labels that include hydrogenated oils or artificial sweeteners are far from their natural states.

HERBAL SUPPLEMENTS

Some herbal supplements can modulate or balance the inflammatory process happening in your body. Taking the supplements and herbs described below might decrease the pain associated with low-back problems. Ask your doctor before taking any supplements. Some medications might interfere with these products, and certain medical conditions might limit the types of supplements and herbs you can include in your diet. Just like over-the-counter and prescription medications, herbal supplements may cause side effects. If you are going to have surgery, you might need to stop taking some of these suggested supplements two weeks before your operation; again, ask your doctor.

Fish Oil

Besides eating cold-water fish, take a daily dose of fish oil. Look for fish oil in the refrigerated section of a supplements store, your local health-food

OSTEOARTHRITIS TREATMENTS

If your back pain stems from osteoarthritis in your facet joints, taking the following supplements may help relieve pain, improve movement, and help repair cartilage in the joints. (Again, ask your doctor before taking any supplements.)

Research shows that taking **glucosamine sulfate** helps repair cartilage, and study patients experienced fewer side effects than participants taking NSAIDs. A study in Portugal showed benefits for 95 percent of the participants with knee osteoarthritis; benefits included less pain while resting, standing, and exercising. Take 1500 milligrams once a day. Make sure you purchase the sulfate form of glucosamine; there is more data supporting its usage than the other form, called glucosamine hydrochloride.

Patients might see more benefits by taking glucosamine sulfate with **chondroitin sulfate**. This supplement may alleviate pain from osteoarthritis and help repair damaged cartilage. Take a daily dose of 1200 milligrams.

Osteoarthritis sufferers may also see symptom improvement while taking **niacinamide** supplements. However, this supplement may cause liver damage and problems with blood sugar. If you wish to take this supplement, do so under strict supervision by your physician.

market, or even in your neighborhood grocery store. In a comprehensive summary study that reviewed the data of several well-done studies, patients who took fish oil for at least three months had less self-reported pain, less morning stiffness of the joints, fewer numbers of painful joints, and were able to reduce their use of non-steroidal anti-inflammatory drugs (NSAIDs). Each day, take two capsules of fish oil with 1000 milligrams of omega 3 fat each. Look for brands that have been independently tested for mercury and other contaminants. Molecularly distilled forms of fish oil are better for you because they are more likely to have had contaminants removed during this process. Look on ConsumerLab.com for brands that have been independently reviewed (see "Resources" at the back of this book). Stop taking fish oil two weeks before any surgery. If you are currently taking a blood-thinning medication, talk to your doctor before starting a fish-oil supplement.

Curcumin

Curcumin comes from turmeric plants. Used for generations in India, curcumin gives curry its yellow color. Of greater importance, curcumin is an antioxidant with anti-inflammatory properties. Take 400 milligrams of curcumin three times a day. This substance absorbs better if you take it alongside a fatty food or if the product is in a gel-cap form. (Supplements in gel-cap form are in an oil base.) Curcumin may work better if you are taking bromelain, the supplement described below.

Bromelain

Bromelain is a mixture of enzymes from pineapple. Studies show this agent lessens inflammation, bruising, and swelling after sports injuries or other traumas. During a 1960 study, seventy-four boxers took bromelain. Within four days, bruising cleared up in fifty-eight boxers, while the rest of the boxers needed eight to ten days for all signs of bruising to disappear. Seventy-two boxers didn't take bromelain. Within this group, just ten participants had no bruising after four days, and the rest of the group needed seven to fourteen days for the bruising to dissipate. For the best results, take bromelain while also taking curcumin. Buy bromelain that is standardized to 2000 mcu's per 1000 milligrams. Take 500 milligrams three times a day, between meals. *Caution*: avoid bromelain if you are allergic to pineapple or if you are on a blood-thinner or have liver problems.

Ginger

Perhaps ginger already flavors some of your dinner entrees. This botanical has anti-inflammatory and antioxidant properties. Take two to four grams of dry, powdered ginger or about a half inch of sliced, fresh ginger daily; you can simply incorporate it into your vegetable dishes. Taking ginger may thin your blood, so talk to your doctor if you are already taking a blood-thinning medication.

Boswellia

The herb boswellia originates from the gum resin of the *Boswellia serrata* tree, which is native to India. Most commonly used as a treatment for osteoarthritis, this herb has anti-inflammatory properties. Look for boswellic acid extracts and take 300 milligrams three times a day. *Caution*: avoid if you have heartburn.

9   WESTERN MEDICAL INTERVENTIONS

YOU DIDN'T THINK YOU WOULD END UP HERE. You're accustomed to trekking up trails full of switchbacks, paddling across lakes, or running up and down a soccer field twice a week. Instead, the very idea of getting out of bed is causing you anxiety. Yesterday you managed to make it through half of your workday before heading home. This morning you are experiencing muscle spasms in your low back, and you have radiating pain coursing through your buttocks and into your right leg.

Before today, easing your low-back pain was simple. You took Tylenol, iced and stretched your back, and spent a few days reducing your activity load, resting more than usual. Clearly, this bout of pain has placed you in new territory. It's time to call your doctor or physiatrist. If she can't help you find an over-the-counter medication to help you get moving again, you'll discuss prescription medications.

Hopefully, your route to healing will end there. But if medications don't allow you to participate in your daily life, what comes next? Injections might alleviate your pain. If they do, you'll move on to physical rehabilitation, participating in therapies we've already discussed in this book.

If your back, buttocks, and leg pain persist, you might start pondering a surgical intervention. Medical treatments for low-back problems have come a long way since the first discectomy surgery in 1934. Major surgeries have become less invasive with shorter recovery times. Still, there is no magic cure-all for lumbar spine pain. When is back surgery the right decision? "I try to keep people away from surgeons unless they have some definite neurologic involvement [numbness, tingling, or weakness, usually radiating into the leg], or if we've tried everything else and they're still having debilitating pain," says family physician Sarah J. D'Heilly, MD, who practices in St. Paul, Minnesota. "Probably upwards of 40 percent of people who eventually get surgery aren't happy with it in the end."

Read on to learn about surgery and if it might be a possibility for your specific diagnosis. We'll also discuss medications, injections, and how to prepare for surgery if you do decide on an operation.

MEDICATIONS 101

Taking medications for low-back pain is just one part of a treatment plan. You should also participate in nonpharmacologic therapies that help alleviate pain and foster healing. Such treatments include any of the numerous therapies we have discussed in this book: physical or occupational therapy, an exercise and stretching regimen, yoga, Pilates, tai chi, acupuncture, chiropractic care, meditation, hypnotherapy, and various forms of massage therapy. Medications can bring temporary pain relief, allowing you to feel better as you participate in non-pharmacologic therapies.

Before taking any medications, it is important to do your research. Even over-the-counter medications have recommended dosages and potentially dangerous side effects. Following are brief descriptions of the most commonly prescribed pain-management medications. Before you start taking any medication, see your doctor for more information.

NSAIDs

Over-the-counter (OTC) pain relief medications are also called *analgesics*. The term *non-steroidal anti-inflammatory drug,* or NSAID, is a catchall phrase for a variety of oral medicines that ease stiffness and reduce inflammation. Commonly used for muscle or soft-tissue injury, these medications are also taken for several low-back pain problems, from disk herniations to osteoarthritis. Topical analgesic creams also can reduce inflammation and ease discomfort. These creams usually contain salicylates, which is the main ingredient in aspirin. If you use NSAIDs or topical analgesic creams for an extended period, possible side effects can include stomach ulcers, or liver and kidney problems. OTC NSAIDs include aspirin, naproxen, ibuprofen; common brand names for some of these drugs are Motrin, Aleve, and Advil. Acetaminophen, with the common brand name Tylenol, alleviates pain as well. For some people, acetaminophen doesn't offer as much pain relief as OTC NSAIDs, but it has the benefit of fewer side effects. (Keep in mind that high doses of acetaminophen can damage your liver.) Follow all the directions and guidelines on OTC medication labels. If OTC medicines don't alleviate pain, ask your doctor about prescription-strength NSAIDs.

COX-2 Inhibitors
Patients typically experience fewer gastrointestinal side effects while taking NSAIDs known as cyclooxygenase-2 inhibitors (COX-2). Take both traditional NSAIDs and COX-2 medications at the lowest possible dose for the shortest period, under a doctor's care. Studies do not support long-term everyday use for these types of medicine for chronic pain. The initial prescription is often for short-term use, combined with other therapies that alleviate pain. You might take these medications for painful flare-ups, or before and after you participate in activities that cause more severe pain. Some studies show that Celebrex and Voltaren and some other NSAID options might increase an individual's risk for cardiovascular events.

Muscle Relaxants
If you have nonspecific low-back pain or muscle spasms, your care provider might prescribe muscle relaxants. Some studies show a benefit in using NSAIDs at the same time. Common brand names of muscle relaxants include Flexeril, Zanaflex, and Robaxin. Muscle relaxants are almost always considered a short-term therapy, usually prescribed for two weeks. Although muscle relaxants often initially help you sleep, sedation and nausea are possible side effects.

Anti-Anxiety Medications
Benzodiazepine or anti-anxiety medications are sometimes recommended for severe pain or muscle spasms. These drugs—brand names include Xanax, Ativan, and Centraz—are discouraged for anything but short-term use. Studies show high rates of physical and psychological dependence. If you take this type of drug, your physician will closely monitor its usage. Side effects can also include tiredness, sedation, and short-term memory loss.

Anticonvulsants and Antidepressants

If you experience chronic nerve pain—including radiating leg pain or other nerve pain in the low back—your care provider might prescribe anticonvulsants or antidepressants as well as NSAIDs. These drugs might alleviate your nerve pain and help you sleep. Common brand names for anticonvulsants include Neurontin, Dilantin, Tegretol, and Topamax. Common brand names for antidepressants are Elavil, Cymbalta, and Prozac.

Steroids and Narcotics

Your doctor might recommend oral steroids for inflamed or swollen nerve pain. Still, no published studies show a benefit for either acute or chronic low-back pain sufferers. There is anecdotal evidence supporting this treatment, though.

Both acute and chronic pain patients are sometimes prescribed narcotic, or opioid, medications for a short time. This type of medication deadens your perception of pain. Opioids can be used when other medications fail to alleviate nerve pain. Side effects are numerous, though, and can include sedation, nausea, cognitive impairment, constipation, itching, and sweating. Long-term use might have a risk for addiction or abuse, so any long-term usage needs to be well thought out and executed with close monitoring by your doctor. Often patients take opioids for just a one- or two-week period.

INJECTIONS

When Minnesota State Patrol Lieutenant Jeff Huettl had two bulging disks and one torn disk, he rested and took pain medications. When his back became stiff and weak, he decided a more extreme treatment was necessary. He had two cortisone injections, with a month of time between the shots.

The first shot had little positive effect, but the second injection relieved his pain. The physical therapy sessions he participated in were also an essential part of his healing process. (See the box "A Home Maintenance Routine," in Chapter 4, for Jeff's full story.)

If, like Jeff, you find that the conservative treatments discussed in this book fail to ease your low-back pain, consider having an injection. Injections are used for disabling pain, meaning you are unable to get out of bed or take part in your normal routine. Ideally, an injection delivers medication directly to the pain area, bringing temporary or sometimes long-lasting relief and enabling you to participate in other treatments, such as physical therapy, stretching, or exercise that will improve your back condition. Different types of injections can alleviate localized muscle pain, relieve muscle spasms, or ease spinal inflammation or specific facet-joint pain.

Be sure to try other treatments for at least four to six weeks before undergoing an injection procedure. "Spinal injections shouldn't be thought of as a mainstay of care," says spine specialist Dr. Stan Herring, spine specialist at the University of Washington in Seattle. "They may have a role as an adjunctive piece, but they do have risks." Any time needle therapy is used, there is a possibility of bleeding, headache, infection, allergic reaction, or nerve damage (although this last side effect is rare).

Surgeons are not the only medical professionals who perform injections; other specialists, such as physiatrists, radiologists, anesthesiologists, and neurologists, use this intervention therapy.

There are various types of injections, each used for a different kind of pain:

Trigger-point injections might alleviate localized muscle pain or break up localized muscle spasms and contractions. A trigger point is a painful area, band, or knot in a muscle. The injection uses a needle to target that trigger point, aiming to relieve the pain. There are several types of medicines used in trigger-point injections, including saline, local anesthetics, or steroids. Trigger-point injections should be performed in conjunction with comprehensive rehabilitation. The goal of an injection is to relieve pain, so you can move and participate in physical types of therapy.

Epidural steroid injections are used to ease spinal inflammation, again allowing the patient to exercise and rehabilitate the back. The needle injects cortisone and anesthesia to the epidural space, the area between the nerve sac and the disk and nerves. Epidural injections can be beneficial for patients with nonspecific low-back pain, sciatica, or spinal stenosis. If a person suffers from low-back pain with no radiating leg pain, statistical data suggests epidural steroids will not alleviate pain. A patient's symptoms should correlate to a specific diagnosis with diagnostic testing, such as an MRI or CT scan. While a doctor might prescribe three injections, the prescription should be reviewed after each injection. You might not need all three injections to achieve your goal. These injections should be part of a treatment plan, including comprehensive rehabilitation. Because of possible side effects, doctors recommend limiting the number of steroid injections given each year. Recommendations vary, but most studies suggest limiting yourself to three injections in a six-month or one-year period. It can take a week to ten days to feel the full benefits of a procedure.

Facet joint injections aim to alleviate pain at specific facet joints, which are the joints at the top and bottom of each vertebra. Facet joints can become painful due to a number of reasons, including osteoarthritis (wear-and-tear arthritis), wear-and-tear on the disks, spinal stenosis, disk herniations, spondylolysis, and sciatica. Facet joint injections work only if the pain is coming from this area. An anesthesia and anti-inflammatory medication, usually a steroid, is used in this type of injection. Like epidural injections, a facet joint injection might take a week to produce the full benefits. Again, this therapy needs to be part of a comprehensive rehabilitation program. Although recommendations vary, most resources suggest limiting facet injections to three times a year.

WHAT ABOUT SURGERY?

Rarely is back surgery or any type of low-back medical intervention an absolute necessity. Medical emergencies that call for immediate spine surgery make up roughly 1 percent of all spine surgeries. (If you have suffered an actual back trauma, you are probably consulting emergency room doctors right now, not this book.) Red-flag diagnoses that lead to quick surgical interventions include cauda equina syndrome, infections, fractures, and tumors. Otherwise, take a deep breath if your doctor recommends any medical procedure, be it a simple trigger-point injection or a fusion surgery. You have time to weigh your options.

Anesthesiologist and pain specialist Mark Matsunaga advises his patients to try nonsurgical interventions if there is any question of where the pain is coming from. "I try conservative management first. Surgery is definitely more costly, the outcomes are not anywhere close to 100 percent, and the patient's anatomy is changed forever," says Dr. Matsunaga, who runs the Comprehensive Pain Center at Howard General Hospital in Columbia, Maryland.

If you are pondering back surgery, keep in mind that only a few medical conditions merit such an extreme intervention. Sometimes, an operation can alleviate pain from a herniated disk, spinal stenosis, or spinal instability. The emphasis in the last sentence is on the word *sometimes*. Although the rate of back surgeries has increased over the last decade, this doesn't mean an operation is a good fit for your specific problem. Despite new technologies and procedures, approach surgical intervention with caution and information. Try nonsurgical therapies first. Medications and injections might relieve pain and ease swelling. Encourage your body's healing abilities with one or more of the numerous options we've discussed in the preceding chapters of this book. Physical therapy, movement therapies, chiropractic care, acupuncture, and meditation are just a handful of the treatments available to you.

CONDITIONS THAT MAY REQUIRE SURGERY

Before you decide on a surgical procedure, you should have tried other treatment options for at least six to twelve weeks. Agreeing to an operation means you have an accurate diagnosis of your specific low-back problem. How do you arrive at such a diagnosis? First, you undergo a thorough medical history and physical exam. Your doctor, spine specialist, or physiatrist will prescribe tests that help pinpoint a diagnosis. There are numerous types of tests. Imaging studies include X-ray, CT scan, MRI, and myelogram; nerve conduction tests include electromyography (EMG) and Somatosensory Evoked Potentials (SSEPs); various blood tests may diagnose autoimmune diseases and rule out other causes of back pain such as kidney stones. While your care provider may order specific tests and explain them to you, it's important that you ask about the significance of the results. How do your results link to your medical history, physical exam, and your daily symptoms, and do these results confirm the need for surgery?

Let's run down the list of conditions that may call for an operation.

Disk Herniations

Our disks—those donut-shaped pads that act as cushions between our vertebrae—degenerate naturally with age. As a disk degenerates, a tear, bulge, or herniation may occur. A disk herniation happens when a sudden increase in the tearing of the outer ring of a disk—the annulus fibrosis—causes the inner nucleus pulposus to actually break through the outer ring.

Disk herniations heal without surgery more than 85 percent of the time. In fact, many people have herniated disks but experience no pain. If you took MRIs of fifty random people with no current or past lumbar spine pain, it's a good bet that more than half of these pain-free individuals would have a bulging disk, and one-fourth of the group would actually have disk herniations. *The New England Journal of Medicine* published a study that looked at back MRIs of people who had never experienced more than a few days of back pain. Sixty-four percent of these individuals had abnormal disks; 52 percent had bulging disks; and 28 percent had herniated disks. If your MRI shows a disk herniation, it may have been part of your anatomy long before you experienced back pain. It's worth exploring the idea that your pain may not be from your disk herniation.

In some cases, however, surgery can relieve the pain caused by a herniated disk. You can consider surgery for this condition if:

- The disk herniation is associated with pain that radiates along your buttocks and into your leg; this is also known as radiculopathy or sciatica. Studies show that low-back surgeries are successful at eradicating leg pain. Studies also show that people who have surgery for disk herniation with leg pain have faster and larger improvement in the short term. However, both people who go through surgery and those who don't are going to have substantial improvement in the long term, and in some studies, the outcome is the same in two years.

- Your physical exam and symptoms are consistent with test findings of disk herniation (or multiple herniations). If your test imaging, such as X-rays and MRIs, doesn't match up with your daily symptoms and your thorough medical exam, surgery probably will not help alleviate your pain. In other words, if your symptoms and the results from your physical exam have no correlation with the disk herniation on your MRI, your pain is most likely from another problem.

Spinal Stenosis and Spinal Instability

Spinal stenosis and spinal instability are two conditions for which surgery might be the best course of action. Spinal stenosis is a narrowing of the spinal canal caused by any number of reasons, including a genetic predisposition, degenerative disk disease, or osteoarthritis of the facet joints. Sometimes spinal stenosis is associated with a disk slippage, called *spondylolisthesis*, or with spinal instability, which simply means an unstable spine. Surgery is called for if the degree of instability or the narrowing of the spinal canal is significant and causing persistent pain, numbness, or weakness in your buttocks and leg or legs.

For spinal stenosis and spinal instability, surgical options include a discectomy, a laminectomy, or a spinal fusion, or a combination of these procedures. Even so, the NASS (the North American Spine Society) recommends spinal fusion surgery only for patients who have failed to improve after six months of nonoperative care and treatments. (If you have major instability and neurologic symptoms that are getting progressively worse, this may not be the case.) If you are only experiencing low-back pain, you can learn to function in a way that diminishes your pain through a combination of therapies, such as medication, physical therapy, meditation, or practicing a movement therapy. If this isn't possible, surgical options should be carefully considered. Remember, surgery rarely clears up all of your back pain—it is much more effective at alleviating buttock and leg pain.

SELECTING A SURGEON

Many highly qualified surgeons perform spinal operations, but not every one of them is the right surgeon for you and your condition. Even if your health insurance policy limits your choices, make every effort to select a surgeon you are comfortable with and who you feel is the most qualified to treat your particular condition. Ask your primary care doctor for recommendations. Talk to family and friends (or friends of friends) who have had back surgery and find out who they used and what their experiences were. Remember that you are in charge of your own medical care—make a careful, informed selection.

It's a good idea to interview at least two surgeons, making each surgeon aware of this good practice. Review each surgeon's qualifications during your appointment. Ask the surgeon how many times he has performed this specific surgery. (An interview process such as this should be a routine procedure for any reputable surgeon.) Most importantly, do you feel comfortable with this surgeon? He might not have time to answer fifty questions, but he should answer a reasonable number and you should feel that he listens to you. The surgeon should see you as an individual, with goals and a set of circumstances that are unique to you. Is surgery—or even a minimally invasive procedure such as an injection—the best possible fit for your life?

Don't Forget to Ask

Before you decide on a surgical intervention, make sure you have all the information you need to make an informed decision. When you are interviewing surgeons, ask the following questions:

- Do my diagnostic tests match the procedure the surgeon recommends? (This is another way of asking if the surgeon knows the specific cause of your pain.)
- What percentage of people have successful outcomes based on my specific diagnosis?
- Is this still an experimental surgery?
- What are the risks, benefits, and possible complications of this surgery?
- What are the pre-surgery preparations and how can I be in the best possible shape for this surgery?
- What will happen before the surgery?
- What happens during the surgery?
- What can I expect post-surgery and during recovery, both immediately at the hospital, and in the weeks and months following surgery?
- Will I need to participate in physical rehabilitation after the surgery?
- What nonsurgical treatments or therapies can I try before agreeing to surgery?

Tell the surgeon you are getting a second opinion. The surgeon you are talking to should welcome another opinion. Avoid any doctor who promises a cure through back surgery. No surgical options for low-back pain have a 100-percent success rate. If you have back surgery and it fails to relieve symptoms, a surgeon might recommend another procedure. Having a poor outcome from one or more back surgeries actually has a clinical name: Failed Back Surgery Syndrome (FBSS).

PSYCHOLOGICAL ISSUES AND SURGERY

Low-back surgery isn't just about the physical aspects of your body. The whole person needs to addressed, including your psychological and psychosocial issues. Sometimes patients experience Failed Back Surgery Syndrome because of psychological and emotional issues.

If you suffer from severe depression, anxiety, or emotional issues, it is best to get support with these issues before you undergo any procedure. A study of childhood psychological trauma, performed at the San Francisco Spine Institute illustrates this point. Eighty-six spine surgery patients were rated for childhood psychological trauma, with risk factors such as physical, sexual, or emotional abuse, neglect, or an alcoholic caregiver. If a person had no risk factors, she had a successful surgical outcome more than 95 percent of the time. If a person had three or more risk factors, there was an 85 percent likelihood of an unsuccessful surgical outcome.

LOW-BACK SURGERIES

There are a vast number of surgical procedures for low-back pain. The type of procedure you have will depend on a specific diagnosis and your surgeon's expertise. Talk with your surgeon about the best options for your particular pain. Assuming that you are comfortable with your surgeon and trust her—and that you have gotten a second surgical opinion—rely on her advice.

Below is an abbreviated discussion of the main types of surgical interventions for the most common low-back diagnoses for active adults. There are numerous other types of surgical interventions. Some of these procedures are for low-back pain typically experienced by older adults, while other interventions are for less common back diagnoses.

Discectomy Surgeries

If you have a herniated disk with nerve pain that radiates into the buttocks and leg, you might be a candidate for a discectomy (that is, having some or all of a disk removed). If conservative treatments fail to alleviate back, buttock, and leg pain, your surgeon might recommend one of several types of discectomies. (Remember, surgical outcomes are more successful for people with low-back pain *and* leg pain. If you experience only low-back pain with no leg pain, look into other pain-management options first.) The most common type of discectomy procedure is a microdiscectomy. During this operation, your doctor removes some of your herniated disk using a microscopic camera and a small incision. With any of these surgeries, your surgeon is trying to alleviate nerve pain caused by the herniated disk.

Laminectomy Surgeries

During a laminectomy surgery, part of your vertebral bone—the lamina—is removed, creating space for pinched nerves in your spinal canal. Sometimes a multiple laminectomy is performed, meaning part of two or more vertebral bones are removed. This type of surgery is most often performed for spinal stenosis (narrowing of the spinal canal).

Spinal Fusion Surgeries

Spinal fusion surgery aims to stabilize an unstable spine, particularly if it is causing pain or deformity. Sometimes spinal fusion surgery is performed to alleviate low-back pain, but it is more effective when it's done to stabilize the spinal column, or when you have both back pain *and* leg pain. Fusion surgery can be performed with your own bone or with donor bone, or with your own bone plus instrumentation. Instrumentation can include materials called

A CAUTIONARY TALE

Dave Helfer, a director of operations at a Seattle-area law firm, was accustomed to dealing with his lumbar spine pain. He was born with a defect in his L5 vertebra that became exacerbated by two stress fractures (L5 and S1) that occurred while he was playing high school soccer. When he turned thirty, he began having sharp pains behind his left knee a day or two after strenuous exercise. Helfer was also experiencing some degree of sensation in his left buttocks and lower back, although nothing notable. After a few months, he saw a neurologist to get an MRI of his back, assuming that the knee pain was originating in his lower spine. "Note that I have dealt with back pain for the majority of my life, so

the back pain was not all that was concerning me—I truly had figured out systems to deal with the pain," says Helfer.

The MRI showed an L5-S1 disk herniation and the neurologist immediately sent Helfer to a surgeon. The surgeon strongly recommended surgery, saying the pain wouldn't resolve without an operation. Since this is a cautionary tale, we'll stop here and point out that Helfer was not experiencing any of the normal sciatic issues—meaning he had no loss of strength, no tingling or numbness, and no contiguous pain from his back down to his leg.

Helfer says the surgery was a success from the standpoint that the "sliver" of herniated disk in the L5-

S1 that was compressing his nerve was removed, but he does not view his operation as successful from any other angle. After the surgery did nothing to ease his knee pain, a knee specialist diagnosed a ligament issue in his knee. A new spine doctor believed Helfer's disk had been herniated for years, and most likely had nothing to do with the knee pain. "As far as pain in my back, it's not all that different than the pain I had prior to the surgery, but now I have to deal with scar tissue and the fact that a knife was put into my back (literally)," says Helfer.

With the help of his spine doctor and a physical therapist, Helfer essentially started over. He tried a steroid injection to calm every-thing down, without success. Taking Neurontin helped, and he has taken this prescription medication for four years. To deal with his back pain, Helfer keeps his core strong by exercising, stretching several times a day, and icing his back every night. He refigured his desk set-up and now uses a kneeling chair. He is always conscious of how he moves, thinking about how he sits, stands, and lifts objects, and how he completes tasks such as getting in and out of his car. "In short, I stick to the program," says Helfer. "It sounds silly, but I try to stay calm. After twenty-plus years of back issues, I know it will pass."

biologics, which are products made from natural sources for medical uses. Discuss the specifics of this type of surgery with your doctor. During a fusion surgery, sections of the backbone are removed and then replaced with one or more of the above-mentioned materials. Over time, these materials should grow together, creating a more stable spine.

Implantable Pain Therapies

Implantable pain therapies are not commonly used. Doctors might talk about this line of treatment for patients with Failed Back Surgery Syndrome (FBSS), or for severe back problems associated with leg pain. As with other surgeries, your diagnosis must match your physical symptoms.

SURGERY PREPARATION AND RECOVERY

Patients who actively participate in their health care have better surgical outcomes than patients who are more passive. You can engage in the surgical process by gathering information about your surgery, asking all of your questions, and feeling comfortable with your surgical decision and your surgeon. Here are other factors to keep in mind when preparing for surgery:

- Try to be in the best physical shape possible for you. Smoking can cause complications, so quitting smoking four to six weeks before surgery is a good idea.
- Discuss with your surgeon the medications and supplements you are currently taking. You might need to stop taking some of them before surgery.
- If you have other medical conditions, such as diabetes or hypertension, meet with the specialists you see for those conditions. You'll want to make sure all of your medical issues are under control.
- Plan for your recovery, with friends and family set up to help with your care after surgery.

- Know what to expect after surgery, from understanding how you might feel to how long your recovery might take.
- Make sure your post-surgery plan gives you enough time to recover, without returning to work or activities too soon.
- Be committed to post-operative rehabilitation.
- Be psychologically ready. You can take part in pre-surgery psychological screening and preparation if you or your doctor thinks this is necessary.

Mind–Body Surgery Preparation

Peggy Huddleston's book *Prepare for Surgery, Heal Faster: A Guide of Mind–Body Techniques* recommends five steps to help people prepare for both surgery and post-operative recovery. Huddleston, a psychotherapist, originally created these tools to help several of her patients have less fear while preparing for their own operations. It's best to start working on these steps two weeks before your surgery, but even if you complete the steps only one day before surgery, Huddleston believes you will still see benefits. Huddleston's five steps are:

1. Relax to feel peaceful. The relaxation CD (or tape or MP3 file) that accompanies her book guides you through an exercise that will put you in a deep state of relaxation. Listen to this twenty-minute CD twice a day.

2. Visualize your healing. Turn your worries into positive healing energy for your back. The relaxation CD will guide you through this process, so you can picture yourself with a healthy back participating in activities that you love. Again, this twenty-minute relaxation CD will guide you through this process twice a day.

3. Organize a support group. Ask your friends and family to think of you with love for thirty minutes before your surgery. Patients who do this report feeling a sense of peace and love wrapping around them like a blanket.

DISK SURGERY STUDY

A study published in 2006 compared the results of patients who have had surgery for disk herniations with patients who opted for nonoperative care. Funded by the National Institute of Health (NIH), the Spine Patient Outcomes Research Trial (SPORT) compared surgery to usual care, meaning the patients and their doctors were free to choose the types of non-surgical care. Each nonsurgical patient received various types of therapy, from epidural steroids, to physical therapy and therapeutic yoga classes. The surgical patients all underwent standard open disc-ectomies. The study rated the patient's recovery for a two-year period. At one year, the individuals who had surgery achieved greater symptom relief, but by the end of the second year, there was no statistical difference between the two groups. After two years, the study showed that it did not matter whether an individual did or did not have surgery.

Some doctors quote this study to recommend an operation for their patients, noting that the surgical patients felt better faster. Other doctors point to the fact that the people who didn't have surgery all received different levels of nonoperative care. Dr. Joel Saar, a disk specialist at SOAR: The Physiatry Medical Group in California, believes that these patients got better because they received specific care, while the nonoperative individuals might have fared better if they had been given a specific regimen of nonoperative care.

4. Use healing statements. Ask a nurse or your anesthesiologist to say three healing statements. As you go under anesthesia, this person says, "Following this operation, you will feel comfortable and heal very well." Toward the end of surgery, this person says, "Your operation has gone very, very well." At the end of surgery, this person says, "Following the operation, you will be hungry for [your favorite white liquid, such as chicken soup]. You'll be thirsty and you'll urinate easily." Each statement should be repeated three times.

5. Establish a supportive doctor-patient relationship. Do this by asking all the questions you have, asking a nurse or anesthesiologist to say the healing statements, and making sure all your needs are met.

A pilot study done at Beth Israel Deaconess Medical Center found that hospitalized patients who were not going for surgery who used Peggy Huddleston's guided imagery tape for twenty minutes twice a day had a reduction in anxiety, used less pain medication, and experienced an improvement in heart rate variability.

You can go through these steps on your own by reading Huddleston's book and using her relaxation CD, tape, or MP3 file. Some hospitals offer surgery-preparation classes based on Huddleston's book, or you can contact her office to locate a health practitioner who will lead you through a one-hour consultation. Huddleston's book is available for purchase online; turn to "Resources" for further information about Huddleston's program.

Following the Huddleston program or using other guided imagery techniques can help you feel more positive about an upcoming surgery. Although numerous studies have shown that patients who have positive attitudes about their operations experience better surgical outcomes, there isn't much information available on preparing your mind for surgery. Huddleston's book and audio program is one option. Meditation that includes guided imagery and visualization is another option. (To learn about starting a meditation practice, see Chapter 6, "Practices for the Mind.")

Post-Surgical Life

After you have surgery, you'll need time to heal. You can complete some of Huddleston's surgery preparation tools post-operatively as well:

- Practice relaxation. Use the *Prepare for Surgery, Heal Faster* relaxation CD, tape, or MP3 file. Alternatively, follow another guided imagery/ visualization audio tape to take you into a state of relaxation for twenty minutes, twice a day.

- Visualize your healing. You can again use Huddleston's audio guide, or try using another guided imagery/visualization audio program for twenty minutes, twice a day.

- Have a supportive doctor-patient relationship. You might wonder if your scar is healing correctly or if the amount of pain you experience is appropriate. Ask your doctor any questions you have and keep the lines of communication open.

It's important to take time to heal, asking family and friends to help care for you. A commitment to your post-operative rehabilitation program will also make your surgical outcomes as good as possible. Of course, surgery is just one piece of the puzzle. You might have pain and discomfort even after you fully heal from surgery. Trying other avenues to healing and pain relief can be beneficial. Read about other therapies, bodyworks, and exercise programs in this book. One or more of them might be a good fit for your lifestyle and your specific low-back issue.

RESOURCES

Acufinder. www.acufinder.org

American Academy of Orthopaedic Surgeons. orthoinfo.aaos.org

American Academy of Physical Medicine and Rehabilitation. www.aapmr.org

American College of Sports Medicine. www.acsm.org

American Heart Association. www.americanheart.org

American Osteopathic Association. 800-621-1773. www.osteopathic.org

American Physical Therapy Association. www.moveforwardpt.com

American Society for the Alexander Technique. 800-473-0620. www.alexandertech.org

American Society of Clinical Hypnosis. 630-980-4740. www.asch.net

Balanced Body Pilates. 800-745-2837. www.pilates.com

Benson-Henry Institute for Mind Body Medicine. 617-643-6090. www.massgeneral.org/bhi/

Center for Mindfulness in Medicine, Health Care, and Society. 508-856-2656. www.umasssmed.edu/cfm

ConsumerLab.com. www.consumerlab.com

ErgoMe. www.ergome.com

Feldenkrais Guild of North America. 800-775-2118. www.feldenkrais.com

Group Health Research Institute. 206-287-2900. www.grouphealthresearch.org

Hellerwork Structural Integration/Hellerwork International. 714-873-6131. www.hellerwork.com

Huddleston, Peggy. 800-726-4173. www.HealFaster.com

International Association of Structural Integration. 877-843-4274. www.structuralintegration.org

Massage Today. www.massagetoday.com

The Mayo Clinic. www.mayoclinic.com

McKenzie Method. 800-635-8380. www.mckenziemdt.org/index_us.cfm

National Center for Complementary and Alternative Medicine. nccam.nih.gov

National Certification Board for Therapeutic Massage & Bodywork. 800-296-0664. www.ncbtmb.org

National Certification Commission for Acupuncture and Oriental Medicine. 904-598-1005. www.nccaom.org

Neutral Posture, Inc. 800-446-3746. www.igoergo.com

PNBConditioning. 206-441-2435; 425-451-1241. www.pnb.org/PNBSchool/PNBConditioning

Prescott, Cathy. www.yogawithCathy.com

PubMed. www.ncbi.nlm.nih.gov/pubmed/

Pujari, M.D., Astrid. www.pujaricenter.com

The Rolf Institute of Structural Integration. 800-530-8875. www.rolf.org

Spine-Health. www.spine-health.com

Spine Universe. www.spineuniverse.com

STOTT PILATES. 800-910-0001. www.stottpilates.com

Stretch Break. www.paratec.com

Strom, M.D., Mark G. www.integrativehealthmd.com

TheraSound. 717-582-4914. www.therasound.com

The Transcendental Meditation Program. 888-LEARN-TM (532-7686). www.tm.org

Yoga Alliance Membership. 888-921-YOGA (9642). www.yogaalliance.org

Yoga Journal. www.yogajournal.com

BIBLIOGRAPHY

Acupuncture. NIH Consensus Statement Online 1997 Nov 3–5; 15(5):1–34.

Benson, Dr., Herbert and Miriam Z. Klipper. *The Relaxation Response.* HarperCollins: New York, 2000.

Bigos, S. J., Battie, M. C., Spengler, D.M., Fisher, L. D., Fordyce, W. E., Hansson, T. H., Nachemson, A. L., and Wortley, M. D. "A Prospective Study of Work Perceptions and Psychosocial Factors Affecting the Report of Back Injury." *Spine* 16, no. 1 (January 1991): 1–6. [Published erratum appears in *Spine* 16, no. 6 (1991): 688.]

Blonstein, J. "Control of Swelling in Boxing Injuries." *Practitioner* 203 (1960): 206.

Brandt, Ryan. "The Owner's Manual: Your Back." *Outside* magazine, March 2007: 51–56.

Buchbinder, Rachelle. "Self-Management Education En Masse: Effectiveness of the 'Back Pain: Don't Take It Lying Down' Mass Media Campaign." *The Medical Journal of Australia* 189, no. 10 (2008): S29–S32. (www.mja.com.au/public/issues/189_10_171108/buc10902_fm.html)

Byström, Sven E. G., Svend Erik Mathiassen, and Charlotte Fransson-Hall. "Physiological Effects of Micropauses in Isometric Handgrip Exercise." *European Journal of Applied Physiology and Occupational Physiology,* 63, no. 6 (December 2004): 405–411.

Cherkin, Daniel C., Karen J. Sherman, Richard A. Deyo, and Paul G. Shekelle. "A Review of the Evidence for the Effectiveness, Safety, and Cost of Acupuncture, Massage Therapy, and Spinal Manipulation for Back Pain." *Annals of Internal Medicine* 138, no. 11 (June 3, 2003): 898–906.

Craft, Peter R., Ann C. Papageorgiou, Susan Ferry, Eleain Thomas, Malcolm I.V. Jayson, and Alan J. Silman. "Psychologic Distress and Low Back Pain: Evidence from a Prospective Study in the General Population." *Spine* 20, no. 24 (December 15, 1995): 2601–2787.

Duke University. *The Duke Encyclopedia of New Medicine: Conventional and Alternative Medicine for All Ages*. London: Rodale Books International, 2006.

Fishman, Loren, and Carol Ardman. *Back Pain: How to Relieve Low Back Pain and Sciatica*. New York: W.W. Norton & Company, 1997.

Gaunt, Angelike M., Stanley A. Herring, and Francis G. O'Connor. "Caring for Patients Who Have Acute and Subacute Low Back Pain." *CME Bulletin,* February 2008: 1–8.

Goldberg, R. J., and J. Katz. "A Meta-Analysis of the Analgesic Effects of Omega-3 Poly-unsaturated Fatty Acid Supplementation for Inflammatory Joint Pain." *Pain* 129, no. 1–2 (May 2007): 210–1223.

Groopman, Jerome. *The Anatomy of Hope: How People Prevail in the Face of Illness*. New York: Random House, 2004.

Huddleston, Peggy. *Prepare for Surgery, Heal Faster*: *A Guide of Mind–Body Techniques* (Second Edition). Cambridge, Massachusetts: Angel River Press, 2007.

Jensen, Maureen C., Michael N. Brant-Zawadzki, Nancy Obuchowski, Michael T. Modic, Dennis Malkasian, and Jeffrey S. Ross. "Magnetic Resonance Imaging of the Lumbar Spine in People without Back Pain." *The New England Journal of Medicine* 331, no. 2 (July 14, 1994): 69–73.

Kabat-Zinn, Jon. *Full Catastrophe Living: Using the Wisdom of Your Body and Mind to Face Stress, Pain, and Illness*. New York: Delta, 2005.

Little, Paul, George Lewith, Fran Webley, Maggie Evans, Angela Beattie, Karen Middleton, Jane Barnett, Kathleen Ballard, Frances Oxford, Peter Smith, Lucy Yardley, Sandra Hollinghurst, and Debbie Sharp. "Randomised Controlled Trial of Alexander Technique Lessons, Exercise, and Massage (ATEAM) for Chronic and Recurrent Back Pain." *British Medical Journal*, 337: a884 (2008). (www.bmj.com/cgi/content/full/337/aug19_2/a88)

Madison, Deborah. *Vegetarian Cooking for Everyone*. New York: Broadway Books, 2007.

Mayo Foundation for Medical Education and Research. *Mayo Clinic Book of Alternative Medicine*. New York: Time Inc., 2007.

McCall, Timothy. *Yoga as Medicine*. New York: Bantam Dell, 2007.

Mehling, W.E., K.A. Hamel, M. Acree, N. Byl, and F.M. Hecht. "Randomized, Controlled Trial of Breath Therapy for Patients with Chronic Low-Back Pain." *Alternative Therapies in Health and Medicine* 11, no. 4 (July–August 2005): 44–52.

Morone, Natalia E., Carol M. Greco, and Debra K. Weiner. "Mindfulness Meditation for the Treatment of Chronic Low Back Pain in Older Adults: A randomized controlled pilot study." *Pain* 134, no. 3 (February, 2008): 310–319.

Myers, Samuel S., Russell S. Phillips, Roger B. Davis, Daniel C. Cherkin, Anna Legedza, Ted J. Kaptchuk, Andrea Hrbek, E. Buring, Diana Post, Maureen T. Connelly, and David M. Eisenberg. "Patient Expectations as Predictors of Outcome In Patients with Acute Low Back Pain." *Journal of General Internal Medicine* 23, no. 2 (February 2008): 148–53.

Olsen, Odd-Egil, Grethe Myklebust, Lars Engebretsen, Ingar Holme, and Roald Bahr. "Exercises to Prevent Lower Limb Injuries in Youth Sports: Cluster Randomised Controlled Trial." *British Medical Journal* 330:449 (February 2005).

Orme-Johnson, David W., Robert H. Schneider, Young D. Son, Sanford Nidich, and Zang-Hee Cho. "Neuroimaging of Meditation's Effect on Brain Reactivity to Pain." *NeuroReport* 17, no. 12 (August 2006): 1359–1363.

Parker, Steve. *The Human Body Book: An Illustrated Guide to Its Structure, Function, and Disorders*. New York: DK Publishing, 2007.

Patrick, G. "The Effects of Vibroacoustic Music on Symptom Reduction." *IEEE Engineering in Medicine and Biology*, March–April 1999: 97–100.

Peters, David and Kenneth R. Pelletier. *New Medicine: Complete Family Health Guide*. New York: DK Publishing, 2007.

Pincus, Tamar, A. Kim Burton, Steve Vogel, and Andy P. Field. "A Systematic Review of Psychological Factors as Predictors of Chronicity/Disability in Prospective Cohorts of Low Back Pain." *Spine* 27, no. 5 (March 1, 2002): E109–E120.

Pizzorno, Joseph and Michael Murray. *Encyclopedia of Natural Medicine*. New York: Three Rivers Press, 1998.

Puetz, Timothy W., Sara S. Flowers, and Patrick J. O'Connor. "A Randomized Controlled Trial of the Effect of Aerobic Exercise Training on Feelings of Energy and Fatigue in Sedentary Young Adults with Persistent Fatigue." *Psychother Psychosom* 77, no. 3 (2008): 167–1774.

Rydeard R., A. Leger, and D. Smith. "Pilates-Based Therapeutic Exercise: Effect on Subjects with Nonspecific Chronic Low Back Pain and Chronic Low Back Pain and Functional Disability: A Randomized Controlled Trial." *Journal of Orthopaedic & Sports Physical Therapy* 36, no. 7 (July 2006): 472–484.

Sarno, John E. *Mind Over Back Pain*. New York: William Morrow and Company, Inc., 1984.

Schofferman, Jerome, et al. "Childhood Psychological Trauma Correlates with Unsuccessful Lumbar Spine Surgery." *Spine* 17, no. 6 supplement (1992): S138–144.

Sherman, Karen J., Daniel C. Cherkin, Janet Erro, Diana L. Miglioretti, and Richard A. Deyo. "Comparing Yoga, Exercise, and a Self-Care Book for Chronic Low Back Pain." *Annals of Internal* Medicine 143, no. 12 (December 2005): 849–856.

Siegal, Ronald D., Michael H. Urdang, and Doulas R. Johnson. *Back Sense: A Revolutionary Approach to Halting the Cycle of Chronic Back Pain*. New York: Broadway Books, 2001.

Sinel, Michael S., and William W. Deardorff. *Back Pain Remedies for Dummies*. New York: Wiley Publishing, Inc., 1999.

Stricker, Lauri Ann. *Pilates for the Outdoor Athlete*. Golden, Colorado: Fulcrum Publishing, 2007.

Tapadinhas, M. J., et al. "Oral Glucosamine Sulfate in the Management of Arthrosis: Report on a Multi-Centre Open Investigation in Portugal." *Pharmatherapeutica* 3 (1982): 157–168.

Tekur P., C. Singphow, H. R. Nagendra, and N. Raghuram, "Effect of Short-Term Intensive Yoga Program on Pain, Functional Disability and Spinal Flexibility in Chronic Low Back Pain: A Randomized Control Study." *Journal of Alternative and Complementary Medicine* 14, no. 6 (July 2008): 637–644.

Toth, M., P.M. Wolski, J. Foreman, R.B. Davis, T. Delbanco, R.S. Phillips, and P. Huddleston. "A Pilot Study for a Randomized, Controlled Trial on the Effect of Guided Imagery in Hospitalized Medical Patients." *The Journal of Alternative and Complementary Medicine* 13, No. 2 (March 2007): 194–197.

Watkins, Kimberly, Stanley A. Herring, and Francis G. O'Connor. "Caring for Patients Who Have Chronic Low Back Pain." *CME Bulletin,* March 2008: 1–8.

Weinstein, J.N. et al., "Surgical vs. Nonoperative Treatment for Lumbar Disk Herniation. JAMA: The Spine Patient Outcomes Research Trial (SPORT): A Randomized Trial." *Journal of the American Medical Association,* 296 (2006): 2441–2450.

INDEX

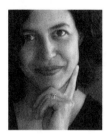

As a nationally recognized internist and medical herbalist, **Astrid Pujari, M.D.,** knowledgeably embraces the best from herbal, nutritional, and mind–body therapies, as well as traditional Western medicine, and safely integrates them into holistic treatment plans. Dr. Pujari received her medical degree from Tufts University School of Medicine in Boston, Massachusetts, and completed her internship and residency training in Internal Medicine at the Scripps Clinic and Research Institute in La Jolla, California. She also completed didactic and clinical training to obtain a four-year medical herbalist degree from the Royal College of Phytotherapy in London, England. She has been certified by the National Institute of Medical Herbalists (NIMH), the leading professional licensing body in Europe, as well as the American Herbalist Guild. She has been selected by her peers as one of Seattle's best doctors and as one of America's best doctors. Dr. Pujari lives in Edmonds, Washington.

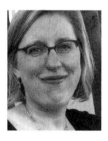

Nancy Schatz Alton is a freelance writer and editor who specializes in health and nutrition topics. She has been managing editor of *Healthy Answers* and *Northwest Table.* Her work has appeared in PCC Natural Market's *Sound Consumer, Seattle Woman* magazine, and online at the food website www.culinate.com and at www.aplaceformom.com. Nancy lives in Seattle, Washington.